PRAISE FOR A NO-NONSENSE GUIDE TO VITILIGO

This ambitious book is about how to help ordinary patients understand and manage their skin condition. Everyone interested in vitiligo should absolutely read it.

— Prof. Torello Lotti

A smart, accessible book that takes a look at the whole body and its environment to understand the disease, treatment tools and protocols, and well worth the price.

— Prof. Robert Schwartz

This is an insightful journey from a patient perspective into the trials and tribulations of living with vitiligo. The author integrates in a flawless form social, medical and psychological burden of living with vitiligo. It is truly the most complete and essential guide to living with vitiligo.

— Prof. Andy Goren

This book is rare. It looks at vitiligo with an insider's knowledge, wisdom and deep caring about patients.

— Ogo Maduewesi, VITSAF

Yan Valle is *the* person to listen about vitiligo.

— Lee Thomas, Fox2 TV

Yan gave over vast amounts of information in a really readable, cogent fashion. This is really a great presentation of a complex topic. ... I am sure that there are hundreds of other diseases, where a guide like this would be really valuable.

— JAMES ADELSON, ZANDERM

I love how easy to understand and comprehensive it is - something definitely lacking in the vitiligo community today.

— ERIKA PAGE, LIVING DAPPLED

A No-Nonsense Guide To Vitiligo is deeply original and well-referenced book. Yan doesn't just list all options for you to choose from, but makes sensible suggestions.

— PROF. KONSTANTIN LOMONOSOV

I must congratulate author on the achievement and contribution he made for public awareness of vitiligo. Its a wonderful book. Both patients and professionals will benefit from it.

— PROF. XING-HUA GAO

Yan explains what's wrong with drug development and why there is still no cure for vitiligo. He also gives a critical, much-needed overview of the effectiveness of various therapies for vitiligo.

— PROF. IGOR KOROBKO

A NO-NONSENSE GUIDE TO VITILIGO

YAN VALLE

VITILIGO TIPS

A NO-NONSENSE GUIDE TO VITILIGO

In this thought provoking and easily accessible book about a neglected skin condition, Yan Valle charts a way towards brighter future without vitiligo. He shares effective principles you too can use to detect early signs of vitiligo, identify potential triggers, develop personalized treatment strategy and manage vitiligo with minimal effort.

Cover design by Stewart Williams

Author photo by Vladimir Bekker

ABOUT THE ADVICE IN THIS BOOK

This book contains the opinions and ideas of its author and is not meant - in either part or entirety - to be a substitute for medical advice. It is intended to provide helpful information on the subject of vitiligo, to be further discussed with the reader's medical doctor. The author is not a licensed medical professional and is not engaged in rendering any kind of professional health service. The reader should consult a competent doctor before applying or adopting any of the ideas expressed in this book. The author and publisher disclaim all responsibility for any liability or risk that is incurred as a consequence, directly or indirectly, from the application of anything covered in this book.

While the manuscript for this book was reviewed by the 501(c)3 non-profit Vitiligo Research Foundation prior to publication, the opinions and thoughts expressed herein are those of the author exclusively.

CONTENTS

TREATMENTS

ACKNOWLEDGMENTS

My deepest appreciation goes to entrepreneur and philanthropist Mr. Dmitry Aksenov and his family, who have provided funding and other support to numerous projects, even before the establishment of Vitiligo Research Foundation. Mr. Aksenov should be acknowledged as one of the key drivers of recent progress in the vitiligo field.

Special thanks also to: Prof. Torello Lotti – a recognized authority in world dermatology – who has been my mentor, colleague and dear friend. Prof. Igor Korobko, a close family friend and fact forager, taught me the value of critical thinking and fact checking. Prof. Robert Schwartz – his charisma, unique presentation style and meticulous attention to minor details have helped forge my writing style.

Just as one generation of researchers borrows knowledge from an earlier one, I have also paid close attention to the many authors who have published on the subject of vitiligo and autoimmunity in general. Reading this book, you may recognize my debt to Professors Andrew Alexis, Xing-Hua Gao, Andy Goren, John Harris, Jana Hercogova, Aliya Kassumkhanova,

Konstantin Lomonosov, Davinder Parsad, Nanette Silverberg, Richard Spritz and Andrija Stanimirovic.

While these people provided the academic framework, others contributed in their own ways to this project. They are too numerous for me to mention everyone, but I could not have accomplished as much without Ogo Maduewesi and Valarie Molyneaux. My gratitude also extends to Martin Sayers – I can't imagine working with a more supportive copy editor, who graciously alerted me to errors and broken English. Thanks to all attendees of my talks in 2012-2017 for listening to my nascent presentations, in which I learned to express myself on truly complicated matters.

Finally, deepest thanks to my family, without whom you would not be reading these words. Under the wise and gentle direction of my dear wife, Julia, I have turned the simple Q&A booklet I started with into a book for the broadest possible audience. My four children were not always enthusiastic about a project that has consumed countless nights and weekends. I thank you for tolerating me and my writing when I should have been relaxing with you. I could have not done this – or even thought about doing this – without all of you.

In many ways, writing is best described by an old Latin saying, "Qui docet, discit" – or "He who teaches, learns." Working on this book was a process of constant learning and discerning, which has been a pleasure. I hope you enjoy reading it and that, when you come to the end, you will have learnt something new about your skin and ways to manage its appearance.

Yan Valle
Toronto, Canada

INTRODUCTION

ABOUT THE BOOK AND ITS STRUCTURE

The book you are about to read is comprised of three sections: Body, Environment, and Treatments. Of course, there is tremendous overlap across the sections, as they are interdependent. In fact, you could think of the three as a tripod, upon which any treatment is balanced. One needs all three to have any sustainable success in treating vitiligo – or indeed any other condition.

However, this book should be enjoyable to read. So don't suffer through the chapters that deal with numbers if you hate math, or with weird names if you hate chemistry. Feel free to skip anything that doesn't grab you and come back to it later. If you decide to flip past something, note it, and return to it later. This is how you *learn from* rather than simply *digest* information. There is a value in the latter, but I hope you'll be actively involved in your skin health management.

I believe that information without emotion isn't retained. If this book were all facts and figures, you'd remember very little.

That's why I've included an ample amount of personal stories and notes, conversations or situations that I was a part of during the past seven years as CEO of VR Foundation. Real-life examples – with names changed to protect privacy – are used to illustrate different vitiligo treatment scenarios, which you can discuss further with your doctor.

I need to emphasize one important qualifier. The advice here is general – it is not optimized for you or for any other particular person. A therapy may be beneficial to one person and harmful to another. The same holds true for nutrition.

WHERE I COME FROM

When I read, I always like to know more about the author or specialist behind the words. It helps me understand the cognitive bias and tools of the person, and to anticipate my learning outcomes. So, here's a bit about me:

My competency in the area you are about to discover evolved from real-life experiences and is built upon a formal education as a computer engineer with a master's degree in business administration. As a professional, I went from nearly three decades in the high-tech and business development sector to become Chief Executive Officer of the non-profit Vitiligo Research Foundation in 2010, upon an invitation from its founder, Dmitry Aksenov – a close family friend.

And as a patient since around six years of age, I have gone through every common pitfall known to a person diagnosed with vitiligo. Misdiagnosis, years of non-treatment followed by bursts of mistreatment – including under-dose and over-dose – treatment dropouts, self-prescription and self-medication, to name a few.

An inevitable side effect of my professional and personal experiences is that I have learned vitiligo inside out, understand the hidden forces driving the disease, tried or familiar with nearly every treatment available, and able to recognize emerging technologies that can bring relief to vitiligo patients.

When challenged with a complicated question, I like to ask myself, "How would I explain this to my mother?" So let's get down-to-earth to make sure you walk away from this book with a clear understanding of your best treatment options and their potential outcomes.

WHY I WROTE THIS BOOK AND WHY YOU SHOULD READ IT

Long before I became CEO of the non-profit Vitiligo Research Foundation, I was reading scientific papers, books and pamphlets to discover more about the stubborn white patches on my skin.

The first one appeared on the knee after skin trauma, very common in soccer playing kids like me, when I was six. When I was 15, new traumas – this time from martial arts practice and shaving – led to more patches. A PUVA therapy prescribed by a dermatologist made me feel sick after three or four sessions, and I had to stop treatment, with no other option in sight.

I stockpiled hundreds of publications on my desk – no e-books back then – only to become increasingly depressed by antagonistic facts and opinions. It took me over a decade to get on top of it all and catch up on the latest developments in the field.

VR Foundation (now known as VRF) started in late 2010. Back then, we assumed that, by pouring money into research, we would discover a silver bullet and vitiligo would be cured. I soon realized it was not going to happen that way. There was much work to do.

So, with support from the VRF Board of Directors, we laid down a solid foundation for other researchers to rely upon and use to build up their programs. A networked biobank was set-up and linked to a centralized bio-informatics system, built specifically for vitiligo research. Grants were provided to leading specialists in five countries.

I have also spent 462 days on the road to date, traveling 1,281,332 miles between 92 cities to talk to hundreds of the world's brightest minds – from traditional healers to Big Pharma CEOs. I kept in touch with eleven laboratories around the world to collect clinical data, and dug deeper into vitiligo and possible cures.

Sharing this information hasn't been an easy task. VRF has embraced an open source concept, which means anyone can use the data, information and knowledge we are collecting. During my years at VRF, we have published 72 quarterly reviews, and contributed to 39 scientific papers and four monographs by prominent vitiligo researchers.

Through a series of master-classes and workshops, we have met with 3,583 doctors, who are now abler to treat their vitiligo patients. We openly share the best practices in vitiligo management, drawn from all over the world – from the Amazon rain-forest to the Dead Sea, to the Himalayas. Yet, this doesn't feel enough when I talk to vitiligo patients and their caregivers, whose minds are cluttered like a bowl of noodles.

Today, medicine is inexplicably tied to finance. The marketing power of social media, celebs, bloggers and pharmaceutical companies undeniably influences our decision-making. I am certain that very few doctors would prostitute themselves for profit, unlike the legions of online vendors and producers of food supplements and cosmeceuticals. Countless self-help books and videos on the Internet promise 'fast cure for vitiligo, *guaranteed*.' This rubbish has worsened skin conditions for the many who, like myself many years ago, have tried these snake oil cures.

Facebook adds to the confusion through mindless link sharing, so that stories of miraculous cures circulate the web. Homeopaths are ready to medicate with their secretive compositions, while experimental treatments are highlighted by respectable media outlets way before they should be.

So, to cut through this mass of information, I have written this book. It's an attempt to consolidate all the scattered scientific evidence, clinical observations and treatment strategies into a single point of reference. My writing is based on hundreds of peer-reviewed publications in scientific journals, work in progress, and countless meetings with specialists.

On this journey through a maze of facts and myths, we'll pause to understand medical jargon and decipher cryptic communications from your doctor. Using the knowledge in this book, you will be able to give your doctor vital information about yourself, to better help him or her offer the therapy *you* need.

Of course, every doctor makes mistakes in diagnosis and treatment. Sometimes, vitiligo symptoms do not readily suggest a clear solution. Other times, there is a range of possible treatments and no single therapy is clearly superior to the others. Doctors and nurses are not infallible, especially in a neglected disease like vitiligo. So, we will review some of the most common mistakes, and how they can be corrected.

I hope this book gives you a solid foundation for your exploration of the vitiligo world. It was written for the layman, though

I believe physicians and caregivers will find it useful, too. It's easy to read over a weekend, yet it is extensively referenced to encourage a deeper investigation into the subject, if necessary.

So settle in, grab some coffee, and get ready to explore the weird, complicated disease called vitiligo.

BODY

PART I

HIDING IN PLAIN SIGHT

1

SPOTLIGHT ON VITILIGO

"**S**top for a second, doc, did you just say there's no cure?" Lee Thomas had dreamt of being on TV since childhood.[1] But now, as vitiligo took hold and his natural brown skin color betrayed him, he could feel it all slipping away. As Lee's hands began to turn completely white, he had to tell his bosses and co-workers about the vitiligo. He feared the worst.

Yet his managers had a surprising reaction: tell your story on the air. So, eleven years after his diagnosis, Lee shared his life and fears with the viewers of WJBK, a local affiliate of Fox TV in Detroit. The Emmy award winner and entertainment guru removed his makeup on the air in November 2005, showing what his skin really looked like.[2] Lee's story got the most feedback the channel had ever seen. Despite a few unpleasant emails and calls, the response was overwhelmingly positive.

Lee's intervention notwithstanding, few people outside the medical professional, and those with the disease, knew the term vitiligo. Then, this obscure skin disease burst into the public spotlight at around 3 pm Pacific Time on June 25, 2009. Online traffic briefly spiked to the maximum capacity of several major networks on the news of Michael Jackson's death and discussion about his recent health condition. News media and celebrity bloggers reported the King of Pop had what they called a rare skin condition – vitiligo – although it wasn't the cause of his untimely death.

The tsunami-like wave of interest in vitiligo re-emerged on August 18, 2014 when Chantelle Brown-Young, a beautiful Canadian model, reached the finals of *America's Next Top Model*. Chantelle's star continues to rise and she is revitalizing the beauty landscape, starring in numerous fashion campaigns in the EU and USA, raising awareness of vitiligo and drawing a million-strong army of devoted fans.

And the ultimate breakthrough in vitiligo awareness happened on Christmas Eve in 2016. Following outcomes of the VRF consensus conference,[3] the United Nations included World Vitiligo Day in its International Calendar of Disability Events.[4]

2

FLAWS ARE BEAUTIFUL

The audience roared their appreciation as the beautiful young woman stepped down from the TEDx stage in London. Chantelle Brown-Young – also known as Winnie Harlow – had thoroughly charmed them with her personality and infectious wit.[5] This high school dropout, who recently grappling with thoughts of suicide, was now a runway queen and inspirational speaker.

Uniquely in Chantelle, vitiligo developed from a blotch on her stomach into a dappled, marble-like effect all over her body, and perfectly symmetrical patches on her face. The overall impression is mesmerizing, and stunningly beautiful.

We met after that TEDx talk at the O2 arena in London to talk about the World Vitiligo Day campaign, celebrated on June 25 every year.[6] I was going to ask Chantelle how we could work together to raise vitiligo awareness, but within a minute of watching her under the blinding spotlights, it becomes obvious there was no need. Chantelle commands attention wherever she goes. Through her army of 1.5 million Instagram followers (at the time of our meeting, it's up to 2.7 million as I write this) she could raise awareness of any subject almost instantaneously.[7] They don't care about her vitiligo diagnosis – they think she's amazing.

And this is part of a growing, and most welcome, trend. Watching major media over the past year or two you might have thought that flaws are becoming a new norm in fashion and TV. People with visual disabilities are campaigning with themes like 'Role Models not Runway Models.' Casting calls for people with 'prominent vitiligo' regularly pop up in my inbox.

Not all those with disabilities suffer from body image concerns and modeling has emerged as a career path for people with all types of flaws. Finding an agent if you are visually different may actually be easier than you think. If you are interested in turning your vitiligo upside down, look up 'disabled model agents' and ask if they are accepting new models. If so, ask if they have open calls, so that you can meet the representative in person. Expect to do some hard work in order to land an agent, and don't take no for an answer. Each agency is looking for something specific, depending upon the needs of the client and what the model has to offer.

There is, of course, still an ocean of neglect and ignorance out there. But any exposure creates a realistic representation of the lives of less-than-perfect people and makes you feel a little less invisible.

3

INVISIBLE PEOPLE

How many people have vitiligo? Let's say we invite everyone with vitiligo to celebrate World Vitiligo Day on June 25 at Mitad Del Mundo – the tall granite monument near Quito, Ecuador, that straddles the equator.[8] With unobstructed views of both hemispheres, this is a suitable place to measure numbers for this global condition, which affects all races, ages, classes and sexes.

With just enough space to breathe, you can fit about ten people on a square meter. On that basis, the amusement park that surrounds the monument can hold about ten million people. But, we've still only accommodated around 10% of our expected guest list. So, we'll start lining everyone up along the equator line, holding hands together. We'll build hypothetical bridges over oceans and tunnels through mountains to make a clean line. Eventually, our imaginary guest line goes around the whole Earth and gets back to Mitad Del Mundo, like a mythological Great Serpent eating its own tale in an eternal cycle of life.

In total, there are approximately 100 million people at our imaginary vitiligo party – about six times the population of

Ecuador itself. If they formed a nation, it would be the fourteenth biggest on Earth, ranked between the Philippines and Egypt.

But this figure is *very* approximate. Even epidemiologists – the detectives of the health world, who study disease occurrence and analyze tons of health related data – have no reliable estimate of the number of vitiligo patients.

Perhaps, the most astonishing thing about vitiligo is how little study on the extent of the disease has been done. Current estimates are rarely based on population-based studies and often are projected from other studies, with different aims, methods, tools and selection criteria. Many were initiated for diseases other than vitiligo. The sample size used in the studies ranged from dozens to thousands of people, thus recruitment bias could have affected the estimates of vitiligo prevalence in unpredictable ways. So researchers try to make sense of the incomplete data they have at hand.

Kruger[9] and Silverberg[10] conducted an in-depth analysis and concluded that worldwide prevalence generally lies within a range of 0.5% to 2%. In a thorough meta-analysis by Zhang and colleagues of 103 studies run in 30 countries over the last 40 years, the prevalence of vitiligo ranged from 0.004% to 9.98%.[11] A projected estimate of vitiligo prevalence in the UK and USA narrows it down to 0.4%, with possible spikes up to 1.5% in certain ethnic subgroups.[12] Finally, there are pockets of India (Gujarat) that are estimated to have an incidence of 8.8% – probably due to genetic or environmental factors.[13]

However, even at the risk of resorting to speculation, I would suggest the number of 'invisible' or unaccounted vitiligo patients mirrors the number of those identified. An undiagnosed vitiligo patient is more likely to be divorced or separated, so lacks the encouragement of a partner to seek help. He or she is more likely to be in a marginal job, with insufficient income to receive proper medical diagnosis and no insurance to receive an expensive treatment reimbursement.

Simply speaking, those who have minor vitiligo will not go to a dermatologist until their skin condition becomes impossible to ignore. With the cost of healthcare in the USA spiraling and growing tolerance towards people with disabilities, discrepancies between hypothetical prevalence, and diagnosed and undiagnosed populations will continue to expand.

VITILIGO IS A PREVALENT SKIN DISEASE, but nearly 100 million people suffering from this condition are seemingly invisible to the healthcare systems of almost every country. While the *true prevalence* of vitiligo is masked from both researchers and the healthcare industry, the *consensus prevalence* number is close to 1% of the population in the USA, and 0.5-2% worldwide.

The number of vitiligo sufferers is also similar to those with hepatitis C, which the World Health Organization has called a 'viral time bomb.' And it is nearly three times higher than the number of people with AIDS, estimated by the WHO at 36.7 million.[14]

Nonetheless, vitiligo is still neglected. In USA, for example, a mandatory Food Allergen Labeling Act helps people with celiac disease to identify dangerous ingredients. Yet – for the twice as many people with vitiligo – there are no warning signs on products that may trigger or worsen their condition. (We will get to that in Part Four, when reviewing *Dangerous Factors and Products* in our households.) Insurance companies turn a blind eye to vitiligo by classifying it as a cosmetic disorder.[15]

MYTH BUSTED: 'VITILIGO IS A RARE DISEASE.' Far from it – most likely, there are more than one or two people with vitiligo in your circle of friends on Facebook.

PART II

VITILIGO EXPLAINED

∽

THE CRUX OF THE PROBLRM

Y ou have a problem, but it's *not* that you are uninformed, misinformed, or lack information. In fact, the opposite is true – patients and caregivers have *too much* information nowadays.

Your real problem is that you cannot interpret the information you already have. And that is hardly your fault. The ordinary person is ill equipped to interpret research papers, clinical data, *pro et contra* arguments and other scientific jargon. Not to mention that half the studies you read about in the news are wrong (but which ones?).[16]

You need explanations from an unbiased expert, to tell you what it all means, to analyze facts and put them in the right order. Only then can you actually use the information you have. However, matters of profound complexity cannot be solved through expertise alone, without the risk of expert's fatal flaw in judgment.

To avoid this trap, we must avoid analyzing *everything* related to vitiligo. This approach will inevitably raise a wave of criticism from experts in fields that overlap with vitiligo, but I suggest we stay focused on the actual broader purpose of information, even at the expense of specific details.

Thus, rather than digging too much into vitiligo pathogenesis and underlying genetics, I will guide you through the key facts established by scientific community to date, put them in context and suggest explanations.

5

BAD AND GOOD NEWS

"Mommy, is it bad?" the little girl asked as she walked out of the doctor's office. "It's just a few spots, right?" Her mother took a deep breath and tried to keep calm. "No, honey, it isn't bad. Daddy and I will make sure you are OK." But her mind was obviously somewhere else.

Mom and her daughter Diana had travelled nearly five thousand miles to meet Prof. Nanette Silverberg at Mount Sinai hospital in New York – probably the fifth or sixth dermatologist they had seen since spots started to appear on the girl's legs and chest a few years ago.

"Could it have been stopped earlier? Maybe, I'm missing something else?" Never-ending questions were rolling through the mother's mind. They walked quietly down the corridor, looking at signs, until they stopped before the lab door. Children with generalized vitiligo need periodic screening for other autoimmune conditions, such as diabetes, thyroiditis, pernicious anemia or lupus, suggests Prof. Silverberg.[17]

A few hours later, the puzzled mom told me Diana had higher than normal levels of androgens, predominantly male hormones – an atypical medical situation for a teenage girl – while other levels were normal. An eye assessment by an ophthalmologist didn't raise concerns for uveitis and retinal pigmentary abnormalities. As I watched the pair leave the hospital, the mom's posture and facial expression were like an *Iron Man* triathlete getting ready for the ultimate challenge.

SURPRISINGLY, the causes of vitiligo are yet to be precisely established. We do know that a triggering event creates stress in the pigment-producing cells of the skin. An over-reactive immune system mistakenly identifies these stressed-out cells as intruders. Specialize cells called T-cells neutralize these 'enemies,' driving progressive skin depigmentation. This can happen to anyone, at any age, in any social group.

About half of vitiligo cases begin in childhood, often popping up in springtime without warning.[18] In white-skinned children, vitiligo spots may remain unapparent until the first suntan of the summer. Sometimes a skinned knee that never regains its pigment is the first indicator of vitiligo. First sightings of vitiligo are common in the diaper area in infancy, and on the face and neck throughout childhood.

THE GOOD NEWS is that vitiligo – upsetting as it can be to those living with it – is neither life threatening nor contagious. The immune system is doing its job too well in vitiligo patients. It kills foreign organisms and pathogens, as well as our own regular cells, including normal and abnormal melanocytes. And because of this hyper-activity of the immune system, those with vitiligo often say they are less affected by common colds.

The bad news is that children with vitiligo may have a higher chance of developing other autoimmune diseases, such as alopecia areata, diabetes mellitus, pernicious anemia, Addison's disease and thyroid disorder.[19] Although rare, hypothyroidism is particularly worrisome in this age group because of its potential impact on growth and health status.

People with vitiligo have a 3x-decreased risk of developing melanoma, which is good news.[20] It seems that vitiligo also has a protective benefit against other deadly skin cancers. As Prof. Nordlund notes: "One of the most mysterious features of vitiligo is the resistance of skin depigmented by vitiligo to producing skin cancers."[21]

Children born to parents who both have the disorder are more likely to develop vitiligo. However, most children will not get vitiligo even if one parent has it. The frequency of vitiligo in the first degree relatives of European whites, for example, is seven percent.[22] In children with focal and segmental vitiligo, there is often no family history of vitiligo or other autoimmune disorders.

6

ELUSIVE MELANOCYTES

So what is vitiligo, anyway? Vitiligo (pronounced *vit-ill-EYE-go*) is a non-infectious, non-life threatening skin disease. It causes loss of skin color and overlying hair on different parts of the body. This happens because of the malfunction of cells that make pigment and hence the color of the skin.

The genes we inherit from our parents primarily determine our skin and hair color. The primordial human skin color is dark. The light color is a genetic mutation passed down through hundreds of generations since our ancestors ventured out of Africa. Thickness of the outer layers, velocity and level of oxygen in blood flow, pigment cells and sunlight exposure also determine skin color. Out of those factors, the single most important contributor is the pigment melanin.

The melanocytes that produce melanin are distributed unevenly across the body. They are located in the basal layer of the skin's epidermis, the iris of the eyes, and also in the hair, nails, inner ear and heart. Melanocytes are branch-shaped, which allows them to transfer pigment granules to other skin cells.

A square millimeter of the skin has somewhere between 900 and 2,000 melanocytes, each about 7 µm in length. There are two times more melanocytes in the same area of the forehead than of the foot.

Through a process called melanogenesis, skin get its 'normal' color – or a long-lasting pigmentation. The purpose of the melanogenesis is to protect the underlying skin layer from the sun's harmful ultraviolet radiation. Dark melanin absorbs a majority of the UV light and prevents skin damage.

The shade of our 'normal' color is very inconsistent. The epidermal melanocyte activity is continuous, while the melanocytes of the hair follicle follow its rhythmical activity. For example, your hair may be blonde as a child, then darken to brown as a teen, and eventually become white in old age.

Exposing skin to sunlight or artificial UV lights catalyze the production of melanin and can result in darker colored skin. This is why light therapy is an essential tool in the restoration of normal skin color.

Several key questions about melanocytes remain unanswered, including the connection between melanocyte depletion and stem cell exhaustion, and the mechanisms and mediators of melanocyte destruction. A complex and poorly understood chain of reactions is controlled by dozens of genes involved in the immune system response and melanogenesis, as recently shown by Prof. Richard Spritz.[23]

When melanocytes become inactive or destroyed for reasons not yet fully understood, skin gradually loses its natural color. This painless process may happen over the course of months or years. It is called vitiligo.

7

UNPREDICTABLE COURSE

Golden Globe and Emmy award winner Jon Hamm says he has developed vitiligo since working on the American TV series *Mad Men*. In an interview with *Rolling Stone* magazine, the actor revealed the disease was non-existent before starring on the AMC drama: "You do have to be mentally acute for a significant period of time, and that becomes pretty draining. I have vitiligo. It's stress-oriented. It comes and goes and waxes and wanes."[24]

Little is known about the impact of psychological stress preceding vitiligo onset, or its effect on the extent of the disease.[25] Nearly half of vitiligo patients say the disease appeared as a tiny blotch and later spread to a wide pattern after severe physical or mental stress. These are called precipitating factors, because they are not the cause of the disease, but induce its appearance. For instance, liver and thyroid diseases could be precipitating factors for vitiligo.

The late Dr. Antonio Salafia, who treated over 19,000 vitiligo patients during his 24-year practice in the poorest neighborhoods of Mumbai, wrote in his chapter of *Vitiligo Q&A*: "In a good number of patients the disease goes on for 3-4 years and then it settles down, with one or two stubborn patches and the clearance of the others. There are also patients where the disease shows periods of stability and then suddenly starts increasing. The natural course of vitiligo is truly unpredictable."[26]

I would add that the course of vitiligo is usually progressive, with phases of stability or even spontaneous reversal. The average remission period after successful treatment of active vitiligo is four years, while the longest was reported by Dr. Aliya Kassumkhanova to be just over eight years. In the book *Vitiligo: A Step-By-Step Guide To Diagnosis, Treatment and Prophylaxis* Dr. Kassumkhanova offers a follow-up protocol to extend the vitiligo-free period.[27]

MYTH BUSTED: 'Vitiligo is a benign skin condition.' On the contrary, vitiligo is a systemic disease affecting the largest body organ and other vital systems.

TIP: Start vitiligo treatment as soon as possible, ideally within the first month or two of spotting natural color fade. This will increase the chance of fast and near-complete repigmentation.

8

DEALING THE GENE CARDS

L ife is a game of chance. Our genes are a deck of cards handed out at birth and every time you shuffle the pack, the outcome changes. It doesn't really help knowing you may be 'at risk' of developing a disease – because you never know if or when you will develop it, or what may cause it.

Even a well-caffeinated person with an advanced degree would have a hard time deciphering genetic research outcomes. Scientists know that some people are genetically predisposed to a specific group of autoimmune diseases – including generalized vitiligo – but do not know why.[28]

Let me take a moment to explain. Our traits – like height or risk of a disease – are not governed by a small number of powerful genes. There are certainly 'core genes' that control vital phases of human existence. Yet they don't work in isolation and are influenced by the body's entire gene network.

This is called the 'omnigenic' model, which basically means that most genes matter for most things.[29] The collective outcome of thousands of weak effects shapes our entire bodies and our health.

Take, for example, a restaurant manager. His or her decisions will define our dining experience, but this manager's life – and thus all decisions being made at work – is continuously affected by the chef and other people in the kitchen, as well as friends and family, patrons, suppliers, etc. If you listed everyone who influences what happens at the restaurant, even in small ways, all of those people would show up on the list. And almost none of them would be individually important for a particular decision.

GENETICISTS ARE RUNNING EVER-BIGGER, genome-wide studies to identify the variants behind most common traits. Historically, even understanding the role of one gene in one disease has been considered a major success. In vitiligo, all the genes that are switched on in a particular type of cell – say, melanocyte – are probably involved in the disease activity.

This might explain why the search for genes responsible for vitiligo has been so arduous. Like a jigsaw puzzle, the pieces of the vitiligo pathogenome are only just beginning to fit together. But most of the identified variants will not yet provide specific leads to a cure, because they exert their influence in incidental ways. It is beyond our current ability to understand how combinations of seemingly hundreds of genes result in a vitiligo patch.

However, there is a lot you can do about your current gene stack. Living in a clean environment on a balanced diet can slash your risk of developing vitiligo, even if your genes are heavily stacked against you. The opposite is also true: an unhealthy lifestyle could scrap the benefit of good genes.

NON-SEGMENTAL VITILIGO IS ASSOCIATED with a tendency to autoimmune illnesses, the most common being thyroid disease.

It roughly equates to the chance of pulling a spade from a deck of 54 cards on the second draw (or 20% vs 25.5%, to be exact)[30]. The chance of getting psoriasis along with vitiligo is similar to pulling a Joker. Chances for endocrinopathies, type 1 diabetes, Addison's disease, lupus, rheumatoid arthritis, and alopecia areata along with vitiligo, is just a bit more than the chance of being struck by lightning. In small studies it was found that vitiligo might negatively affect hearing[31] and eyesight.[32] Researchers also associate vitiligo with celiac disease, Crohn's disease and ulcerative colitis, among others.

MYTH BUSTED: 'Vitiligo is contagious.' No way. Bad melanocytes cannot jump between people.

TIP: Share your concerns about possible health complications with your doctor, using a medical term – 'comorbidities.' He or she will be able to create a screening protocol to watch for early signs.

PART III

DIAGNOSING VITILIGO

~

9

A TWO-FACED DEITY

I n ancient Roman myth, Janus is the god of gates, transitions and time. He is usually depicted as having two faces, presiding over all beginnings and transitions, whether abstract or concrete, sacred or profane.

Prof. Torello Lotti and colleagues argue that vitiligo, like this ancient deity, has two distinct faces:

- **Segmental**, also called unilateral or one-sided vitiligo, happens on one part of the body. It often starts at a young age and usually stops spreading after a year. The cause may involve the nervous system.
- **Non-segmental**, also called bilateral or generalized vitiligo, may appear on all body parts, especially areas that are bumped or rubbed frequently. These patches often extend slowly over time if left untreated. The cause may involve the immune system.[33]

An early distinction between these two basic types of vitiligo is very important in predicting disease activity and choosing the right treatment. The Vitiligo European Task Force breaks these types down further into subtypes, but I won't trouble you with these, as they are not easily understandable.[34] Here's what you need to know about segmental vs. non-segmental vitiligo:

As THE THEORY GOES, *segmental* lesions stay on one side of the body, rarely crossing the midline. Yet, *non-segmental* vitiligo can begin initially, and often stays localized, on one body part for long periods.[35]

Segmental vitiligo usually starts in childhood, at the average age of fifteen.[36] The lesions develop rapidly, within one to four years, in a localized area and then remain stable for life. This type of vitiligo responds poorly to medical treatments, like phototherapy and medications, but responds very well to micro-surgical methods, with a lower risk of recurrence.

In contrast, non-segmental vitiligo affects multiple body parts, often remarkably symmetrical – as seen in the model Chantelle Brown-Young – with unpredictable periods of activity. A small number of patients go from having dark skin to having totally depigmented skin and hair in a period of months. The late Dr. Lerner called it 'veloce vitiligo,' or rapid vitiligo.

NOTE: As Prof. Harris wrote in his comment to an early draft of this manuscript: "We are trying not to use the term 'non-segmental vitiligo' anymore, since it defines the most common form of vitiligo. Generally, we've started saying that segmental vitiligo is a subtype of vitiligo."

10

FIRST SIGNS ON VITILIGO

Vitiligo signs vary considerably from person to person. It is more pronounced in people with dark or tanned skin. Some may only acquire a handful of white spots that develop no further. Others develop larger lesions that join together and cover significant areas of the skin.

Vitiligo extent also varies considerably depending on the place of birth and residence, especially early in life. For reasons not yet clear, those born in the U.S. have a greater chance of extensive vitiligo that covers over 25% of the total body area, compared to the rest of the world.[37]

Initially, vitiligo starts as a simple spot, a little paler than the rest of the skin. As time passes, this spot gradually becomes lighter until it turns milky white. The shape of these patches is completely irregular. Occasionally, it may have an inflamed border with a red tone, resulting in itchiness.

Vitiligo also favors sites of injury, such as cuts, scrapes or burns. This is called the 'Koebner phenomenon' and is notoriously difficult to treat.[38] Often, this is a first sign of vitiligo. A halo nevus – a mole with a white ring or 'halo' around it, usually on the trunk – can also be an early warning sign of generalized vitiligo. It is often seen in young children with early stage vitiligo.

Hairs overlying vitiligo patches may also lose pigment and appear white. This is called leucotrichia, sometimes referred to as poliosis – a broader definition for a patch of white hair. But the brown spots that appear around hair follicles in the depigmented skin are a good sign of re-pigmentation process and prognostic factor for treatment.

Other than the appearance of the spots and occasional itchiness, vitiligo does not cause any discomfort, irritation, soreness, or dryness of the skin. Yet, patients often report itching around lesions.

VITILIGO OR LEUKODERMA?

Not every white patch is a sign of vitiligo. Broadly speaking, loss of skin pigmentation is called leukoderma. Vitiligo is a specific type of leukoderma and is often, though incorrectly, used interchangeably with the term leukoderma.

There are many potential causes of leukoderma. Thermal burns, inflammatory skin disorders like psoriasis, or bacterial infections like leprosy may cause a reversible loss of skin color. Genetically determined diseases like piebaldism can also create distinctive patterns of milky white skin and hair, which can be mistaken for vitiligo. Skin color restoration in these conditions is not an easy task and requires elaborate techniques, with a low success rate.

Furthermore, loss of skin color can be caused by contact with chemicals known to destroy the skin pigment cells. These are usually chemicals found in the workplace, but also in certain cosmetic products. This skin condition is known as chemical, or contact, leukoderma. We'll dig deeper into this in the following chapters.

DIAGNOSTIC TOOLS

L oss of pigment from the skin is the hallmark of vitiligo, which is normally easily distinguishable in dark-skinned people. It may, however, be very difficult to recognize vitiligo in fair-skinned people because the difference in color between normal and abnormal skin is minimal.

A well-trained dermatologist should be able to distinguish vitiligo from contact leukoderma or more than twenty other conditions with similar skin appearance. Vitiligo is often diagnosed based on physical examination, assisted with a Wood's lamp and tests, whenever necessary.

Medical History and Examination

Information about your past and current health may help your doctor make a correct diagnosis. He or she may ask you when white or lighter patches of skin first appeared and whether they affect several parts of the body or remain in one location. Your doctor may also ask if you have been diagnosed with an autoimmune disorder, such as hypothyroidism or type I diabetes, and if any of your family members have a history of vitiligo or an autoimmune condition.

Your dermatologist should also perform a thorough examination of your skin from head to toe, to identify the type and extent of your vitiligo and map where depigmentation appears and the patterns it forms.

VRF has put a very useful tool online that helps patients get ready for a doctor's visit.[39] You can answer simple questions in your web browser anonymously, then print out or email it to your doctor.

Wood's Lamp

If you've ever been to a nightclub, you've already encountered the simplest diagnostic tool for vitiligo. These are the 'black light' tubes that emit UV light with a bluish glow, which are often used to check fluorescent re-entry stamps or to highlight design elements in the dark. Black light is also used in counterfeit money detectors and during the examination of crime scenes. Clothing lint often shines bright white under black light.

In medicine, this type of light is called a Wood's lamp. It emits on a 320-450 nm wavelength, which is completely invisible to the human eye – hence the name 'black light'. A Wood's lamp glows violet in a dark environment, because it also spills some light into the violet part of the electromagnetic spectrum. This light is harmless and will not damage your skin. However, do not look directly into a working lamp for more than a few seconds.

A Wood's lamp diagnosis takes place in a dark room, with the lamp held 4-5 inches (10-13 cm) away from your skin. Normally your skin will not fluoresce, or shine, under the lamp – but patches of vitiligo or other conditions will be easier to see.

Healthy skin shows a slightly blue color, oily skin looks yellowish, and dehydrated skin looks purple under UV light. Some skin diseases give off particular colors, like:

- golden yellow (tinea versicolor),
- pale green (trichophyton schoenleini),
- bright yellow/green (microsporum audouini or m.canis),
- aqua green to blue (pseudomonas aeruginosa),
- pink to pink/orange (porphyria cutanea tarda),
- pale white (hypopigmentation, in general), or
- purple/brown (hyperpigmentation, in general).

Skin lesions with vitiligo will appear bright white or blue/white, depending on the progression of the condition. Drugs on the skin surface, such as tetracyclines and mepacrine, fluoresce after oral ingestion. Gupta and Singhi put together a good review of other possible uses for a Wood's lamp.[40]

If you know your doctor is going to examine you with a Wood's lamp, it is best to not wash the area, and not apply any cream or deodorant to the skin to avoid inaccurate – called 'false negative' or 'false positive' – results.

Prof. Silverberg has reported a 'false highlighting' case, when a 5-year-old boy had painted his face with highlighter, producing enhancing lesions under a Wood's lamp.[41] She says that most children are covered in false positives, such as milk moustaches, sock lint and magic markers.

Other common sources of misdiagnosis are the bluish or purplish fluorescence produced by ointments containing petrolatum, green fluorescence through salicylic acid containing medicaments, and light reflected from an examiner's white coat producing a light blue fluorescence.

Blood Tests

Occasionally, your doctor may recommend some tests to get more information about a possible autoimmune response related to vitiligo or associated diseases. (Remember this term 'comorbidities' and the doctor will certainly appreciate you doing homework.)

Tests may be recommended, if:

- Your doctor suspects other underlying or comorbid conditions – like thyroiditis or diabetes – that require a blood test.
- A patient (usually a child) has extensive abdominal complaints like bloating and cramping. This would require screening for celiac disease.
- To rule out the possibility of a form of skin cancer, which may cause white patches due to malfunctioning melanocytes. This would require a skin biopsy.

If your doctor is also involved in research or clinical trials, he or she may need to get more information about how the vitiligo affects your skin. This would require a skin biopsy or a blood test, after doing all the necessary paperwork that comes with it.

At a later stage, some vitiligo treatments may require checking levels of vitamin B_{12}, interleukin and specific antibodies. In preparation for microsurgery, tests may also include a complete hemogram, bleeding and clotting time, and blood sugar. When low vitamin D levels (25-hydroxyvitamin D <15 ng/dL) are detected in children older than three years and adults, this demands screening for other autoimmune diseases.

Skin Biopsy

A skin biopsy is a simple medical procedure in which a small sample of your skin – the size of a grain of rice – is taken and tested in a laboratory. It can definitively tell the difference between missing melanocytes, which indicates vitiligo, and melanocytes that are malfunctioning for another reason.

The procedure normally involves local anesthesia to numb

the biopsy site, before the sample is taken and the wound covered with gauze. It usually takes about ten minutes and you'll normally receive results in about a week, although some tests can take longer.

MYTH BUSTED: 'Vitiligo will soon take over my body.' Not necessarily true: there is a good chance it will confine itself within one body part for many years. As Prof. Silverberg says, "How it starts is how it finishes." The severity of the generalized disease can be predicted by the treatments received in the first six months to one year.

ENVIRONMENT

PART IV

DANGEROUS FACTORS AND PRODUCTS

~

13

WHY THE HECK HAS NOBODY TOLD ME THIS BEFORE?

Think, if you will, of the journey of freshwater. As you move upstream, you get to its source or – more likely – to a complex watershed that creates the lakes, creeks and rivers that bring it down to the oceans. If we look at vitiligo from the Mitad Del Mundo perspective, it quickly becomes clear that both *upstream* and *downstream* solutions are needed to solve this problem.

When we're looking at vitiligo from the dermatologist's viewpoint – capturing signs and symptoms and prescribing topical treatments – we're moving downstream with the disease. But if we were to use the upstream approach, we could explore ways to eliminate the possible root causes: to remove products from our living environments that make us sick in the first place.

Upstream solutions are almost always more effective, as they can get to the heart of the problem. And in doing so, they often bring many more problems to light, which are often systemic, complex and challenging. They open up the opportunity to create new treatments for many diseases. But they can also trigger a tsunami of negative reaction from the biopharma industry, insurance companies and – further down the ladder – the mid-level managers worried about their paychecks.

As explained in the following pages, there are many factors that can cause or worsen one's vitiligo. Most, but not all, are easily avoidable. Worse, these factors affect multiple body systems simultaneously, often creating an avalanche-like chain of events and causing key organs to malfunction.

Now your totally understandable question is probably: "*Why the heck has nobody told me this before?*" Well, the answer is that most doctors are not specifically trained to look upstream, and certainly none are paid to do so.

So, let me take you upstream to where vitiligo commonly begins, to see what we can find there.

14

STRESS IS THE MOST COMMON TRIGGER

Nearly three quarters of the population carry genetic traits than can cause vitiligo, although it develops properly in only 0.5% to 4% of all people, depending on the region. This incurable disease typically manifests itself before the age of 50, and equally affects all sexes, races, and social groups.

Researchers know the cause is pre-wired in your genes, just waiting for a bad luck moment. In about half of all cases this can be a specific trigger or an unfortunate combination of benign conditions. In the other half, the cause of vitiligo remains unknown.

On the outside, severe sunburn, physical skin damage, prolonged contact with certain chemicals, hair dyes or even common home care products may induce or worsen vitiligo. Although extremely rare, cancer radiation therapy may also trigger generalized vitiligo.[42] As seen earlier in this book, variation in rates for extensive vitiligo indicate that regional environmental risk factors play an important role in developing vitiligo.

On the inside, psychological stress is the most frequent trigger for vitiligo.[43] Prolonged lack of sleep and undue stress –

for instance, during final college exams – is repeatedly reported as a precipitating factor for vitiligo. Hormonal changes during pregnancy, delivery and menopause may also be the culprit, as can excessive pressure and friction from lingerie, shoes, or sporting equipment – even many years after the contact.

Parasites and chronic gastritis that impair absorption of vital elements by the digestive system may also precipitate vitiligo. This observation has been frequently reported by doctors in Central Asian countries, including Kazakhstan, Kyrgyzstan, Tajikistan and Uzbekistan, but it is not common in North America.

15

CHEMICAL TRIGGERS IN THE POOL

The Winter Consensus Conference on Dermatology is held once every four years.[44] In December 2012 over 150 high-profile delegates – including two Nobel Laureates – gathered in the sleepy town of Kitzbühel in Austria to focus their undivided attention on vitiligo. As chair of the Roundtable and CEO Task Force, it was my job to select keynote speakers for my section. One of the most experienced and – as often happens – the least known to the public, was the late Dr. Antonio Salafia. He had a lot to share.

Dr. Salafia reported a disturbing case. Three unrelated young girls and two boys of Indian origin developed vitiligo after using a swimming pool at their posh neighborhood in Mumbai on a daily basis for two or three months. Dr. Salafia had repeatedly stressed that chemically induced vitiligo is not a rarity, but a common happening in the developing world.

IT IS NOT unusual for water in public pools to go unchanged for years, especially where water is scarce. On average, a decently maintained, commercial pool in the U.S. with a 220,000-gallon capacity (830,000 l) contains around 20 gallons (75 l) of urine. In a residential pool 20-by-40-foot (6 by 12 m), five-feet deep (1.5 m), that would translate to about two gallons (or 7.5 l) of pee.

The only way to remove pee and other bodily fluids is to replace all the water. But clean water is expensive in many places – from the highlands of India to the California coast.

Instead of replacing pool water on a regular basis, many operators prefer to just add water and chlorine. Over months and years, as more chlorine meets more sweat, body oils and urine in the water, it creates a number of potentially toxic compounds, collectively called disinfection byproducts. These can include anything from chloramines, which give well-used pools that infamous odor, to nitrosamines that can cause cancer, to cyanogen chloride, which is classified as a chemical warfare agent. And the longer water sits in a pool, the worse it gets.[45]

STRICTLY SPEAKING, chemically induced loss of skin color should be first considered as contact leukoderma. The main chemicals and their derivatives that have been known to cause loss of skin color include:

- p-phenylenediamine (also known as para-phenylene diamine or PPD),
- para-tertiary butylphenol (PTBP), and
- monobenzylether of hydroquinone (MBH).[46]

PPD and PTBP are also known by many other unpronounceable names – check them on the Contact Allergen Database.[47]

Avoidance of these chemicals usually results in the recovery of skin color, especially if there is no family history of vitiligo. However, further extension of the depigmented area indicates a genetic tendency to vitiligo.

For your own safety at work, you can ask for Safety Data Sheets, which in many countries are required for all chemicals and substances you may come into contact with in your job.

16

DANGEROUS PRODUCTS IN YOUR HOME

Your home is stuffed with products known to be toxic, carcinogenic, and hormonally disruptive. I'm not talking about the necessary evil – household cleaning items. They are plastered with warning signs and recommendations for safe use. With proper precautions, the damage to your health is transient and recoverable – unless you are allergic to specific compounds.

I mean body washes, shampoos, and skin care products, which contain countless chemicals that – unlike drugs – are not tested or monitored. To help people screen their environment, the United States Department of Health and Human Services maintains a Household Products Database detailing the potential health effects of over 18,000 consumer brands.[48]

Yet health-conscious shopping remains a challenging task. Firstly, you won't find warning labels on all potentially harmful products. Secondly, there's no high-profile campaigns to tell us what's safe and what's not. Thirdly, many dangerous ingredients are disguised under different names – known only to health freaks, chemistry students and professionals. Finally, not all products are equally dangerous to all people.

IF YOU ARE at risk of developing vitiligo or are prone to contact allergy, try to avoid products containing para-phenylenediamine (PPD) and para-tertiary butylphenol (PTBP). These products are common at low-cost stores, markets and street vendors, but can also be found in these beauty products:

- Permanent or oxidation type hair dyes, which are usually recognized by coming in a two-bottle preparation. Ask your hairdresser to switch to vegetable rinse hair dyes instead.
- Skincare creams with these words on the label: 'whitening', 'lightening', 'brightening' or 'anti-pigmentation' (more on this follows in the *Snow White Syndrome* chapter).
- Sunscreens, lotions and creams with para-aminobenzoic acid (PABA).
- Dark colored lipsticks, lipliners and eyeliners from dubious brands.

You should also be careful with:

- Glued leather goods, such as handbags, wallets, belts and watchstraps. (*Sewn leather goods are a safer alternative.*)
- Black socks and other footwear from a questionable supplier.
- Sponge rubber insoles in athletic shoes. (*Always wear socks in your sneakers, and change them frequently to avoid sweat from building up and dampening the shoes. Moisture causes breakdown of chemicals and release of the PTBP allergen, thus allowing contact with skin.*)
- Rubber chappals, flip-flops or jelly shoes. (*Try to avoid*

getting these wet or soaked by water, for the same reason as above.)

- Plastic bras or neck wallets. Also, plastic bra stripes are well-known causes of leukoderma in India.
- Adhesive used to stick a Bindi dot.
- Azo dye in alta – a scarlet-red solution used by some women as a cosmetic to color their feet.
- Mercuric iodide-containing 'germicidal' soap.
- Temporary black henna tattoos (*more on this in the next chapter*).

Industrial items with PTBP include printing inks, motor oil additives, fiberglass products, plywood, masonry sealant, insecticides and commercial disinfectants. Medical items with PTBP include hearing aids, prosthesis and athletic tape.

Talk to your doctor or dentist about elevated risk of vitiligo if you are receiving a local anesthetic, such as aminoester, benzocaine and procaine, or are getting tuberculosis treatment with para-aminosalicylic acid. Although rare, drugs like imiquimod and amyl nitrite can also cause vitiligo, localized to sites of exposure.[49]

17

TEMPORARY TATTOO, PERMANENT DAMAGE

A 10-year-old British kid returned from his Spanish vacation with a cool souvenir decorating his forearm – a temporary black henna tattoo of a pirate skull-and-crossbones. However, very soon his skin erupted in a painful, swollen rash along the tattoo's outline. The child was treated with antibiotics and topical creams and after two days, says a BMJ report,[50] his skin condition improved and the inflammation went down. However, a vitiligo-like loss of normal skin color inside the tattoo area was apparent weeks later.

Black henna tattoos are different from the more popular red henna tattoos. The latter is a traditional body decoration for special occasions throughout Africa and Asia. It has nothing to do with another kind of body art – permanent tattoos.

Natural henna is made from a flowering *Lawsonia inermis* plant. When applied directly to the skin, henna can leave a brown or reddish-brown tint. Red henna skin ornaments are generally safe and typically fade in one or two weeks.

To satisfy travelers' insatiable appetite for instant entertainment, street sellers came up with black henna temporary tattoos. In order to make temporary tattoos look more like a real tattoo, dry quicker and last longer, they mix natural red henna with the chemical compound para-phenylenediamine – also known as p-phenylene diamine or PPD.

Varying amounts of PPD may be found in black henna ink. A safe level for skin and hair products is considered less than 0.2% and 2% concentration, respectively.[51] However, some have been found with a 30% concentration mix. Often kerosene or petrol is also added to speed up the color intake by the skin. The mix is then painted or airbrushed onto the skin.

The results can be devastating. A skin reaction may appear from a few minutes up to 14 days following application. The reaction usually slowly resolves itself. However, an improper PPD mix may cause a loss of consciousness, respiratory distress, severe skin reactions or permanent vitiligo-like lesions. PPD can also sensitize patients to other allergens for life, inducing hypersensitivity to natural rubber latex and PABA sunscreen. Treatment generally involves the use of topical or oral corticosteroids, antibiotics and antihistamines.

Like temporary tattoos, permanent tattoos have their own serious health risks. There are many reasons, besides the aesthetic, for tattooing oneself – such as an initiation rite, or medical reconstructive procedure. Check Part Ten for possible use of tattoos as a cosmetic camouflage for vitiligo.

MYTH BUSTED: 'It's just for fun, everyone does this.' Just because a tattoo is trendy, doesn't mean it's risk free. Think before you ink and avoid black henna temporary tattoos, period.

TIP: Use the Household Products Database to check your beauty cabinet and cleaning box for potentially dangerous products.

18

SNOW WHITE SYNDROME

I was amazed by a report in Asian Scientist that revealed sales of skin whitening creams in India were far outstripping Coca-Cola.[52] Today, whitening products comprise nearly 75% of the cosmetic market.

In our culturally constructed world, skin color is loaded with socially defined meaning. Obsession with skin color has a long history in Asia, dating back to the Vedic times, when *apsaras* – mythological celestial maidens – were said to be sent to distract a spiritual master from his ascetic practices with their fair skin and artful dancing. In Indian tales, protagonists are typically fair-skinned and depict virtue and goodness, while antagonists are described as being dark-skinned. British rule in India further propagated colorism, as the upper castes typically had fairer skin and did not indulge in outdoor activities like the lower castes.

Nowadays in Asia, fair skin is coveted for its perceived beauty, as propagated by the stereotypes peddled by the movie and marketing industries. This phenomenon is called 'Snow White syndrome' and is endorsed and fueled by male and female celebrities alike.

SKIN LIGHTENING IS A WELL-ESTABLISHED PROCEDURE. Many of the active ingredients found in consumer-grade creams are successfully used by dermatologists to treat hyperpigmentation. Global brands typically play safe – so concentrations of active ingredients in over-the-counter products are too low to be dangerous (or useful) for most people. Local brands are getting a bit more aggressive with melanocytes, but knock-off brands will use double and who-knows-what concentrations for immediate results. Over-use of these products without a dermatologist's supervision can cause severe consequences.

But skin bleaching components are everywhere, often unacknowledged or hidden under fine print: in lotions, moisturizers, soaps and shampoos. The cost of these products ranges from $150 per tube down to 50 cents, making them both desirable and accessible to almost everyone. Unsurprisingly, it's causing problems: India has one of the highest rates of vitiligo prevalence in the world!

WOMEN IN NIGERIA are raising the bar even higher. The World Health Organization reported that a whopping 77% of Nigerian females regularly apply skin bleaching products.[53] 'Fanta face, Coca-Cola legs' has become part of the lingo, denoting people who lighten their skin on the upper body only.

In Abuja, the Nigerian capital, I saw a store's cosmetics aisles filled exclusively with 'fairness' products. There were many brands to choose from, boasting 'whitening', 'lightening', 'brightening', 'freshening', 'anti-pigmentation', 'anti-dullness' and even 'illuminating' properties.

A 2013 SCANDAL involving skin-whitening products from Kanebo, a major Japanese cosmetics company, showed that no customer is safe from an occasional exposure to harmful substances. Reports of white blotches from thousands of customers forced the company to recall 54 of its products from five brand lines containing an ingredient called 'rhododenol' (4-(4-hydroxyphenyl)-2-butanol). Symptoms included "depigmentation in three or more areas of the body," "depigmentation in an area of at least 5 cm" and "clearly visible depigmentation in parts of the face."[54]

Almost 20,000 consumers have been confirmed as suffering from vitiligo-like symptoms – of which almost 12,000 have fully or nearly recovered. The company has reached settlements with 15,000 people for an undisclosed amount of money, likely to be tens of millions of dollars.

THE WORLD HEALTH ORGANIZATION report noted the active ingredient in these products — mercury salts used to inhibit melanin formation — can cause poisoning, kidney damage, reduce the body's natural ability to fight bacterial and fungal infections, and lead to memory loss and psychiatric disorders over a long period of exposure.

Some of these ingredients — like hydroquinone or steroids — are banned for use in cosmetics in the USA and European Union, although available as a medication. Misuse of hydroquinone can paradoxically lead to a blue-black darkening of the skin called ochronosis. Prolonged use of steroid creams can cause skin-thinning, acne, stretch marks, and increased skin infections.

The bootleg double-strength versions that promise 'fairness in four weeks' are particularly hazardous. People trying to avoid color discrimination can find themselves permanently trapped in the vitiligo camp.

But this desire to change skin color works both ways. In North America and Europe, tanned skin is becoming more popular, as it is associated with a life of wealth and leisure. An obsession with caramel-colored skin is linked with a meteoritic rise in skin cancers in Europe.

Needless to say, the arguable beauty benefits of skin lightening and darkening are *far* outweighed by the potential dangers.

MYTH BUSTED: 'You can detox from vitiligo.' While certain chemicals can induce or worsen vitiligo, it's not caused by a toxin that can be removed from your system.

PART V

THE PROBLEM WITH DRUG DEVELOPMENT

~

19

WHY THERE IS STILL NO CURE FOR VITILIGO?

Hostage events have been some of the most difficult cases for law enforcement, and the most spectacular and newsworthy happenings for mass media. And, since the time of 9/11, I can't stop thinking of the parallels between the complexities faced by law enforcement and those that face the immune system.

How do you begin to distinguish terrorists from hostages from security personnel on board a plane traveling at 540 miles per hour at an altitude of 33 thousand feet (or 870 km/hr at 10,000 m)? How do the authorities prevent further damage on the ground, while protecting hostages on the plane?

The challenges faced by the immune system are similar. It too must selectively target and destroy unwanted elements, protect its own, and make a safe delivery of the precious load, without creating too much disturbance in the process.

Perhaps the answer is build a profile of every possible dangerous or abnormal element — thus preventing them from hijacking modes of transportation? That's exactly what law enforcers try to do. And the same is also the basis for much vitiligo research, but there are many problems:

Firstly, we don't always know why and how 'normal' starts to become 'abnormal'. Because the abnormal disease-causing cells in autoimmune diseases are also involved in many normal processes, we can't target them at will without creating unintended side effects.

Consider this simple fact: there are around 200 types of cells in the body. But then, there are subtypes upon subtypes. Each subtype can exist in many different states based on its tissue and environment. To complicate matters further, some types of cells can transform into others.

The second problem is that existing therapies aren't good enough at selective targeting inside a complex organism. So most therapies either treat symptoms only – without curing the disease – or destroy both the disease and specific immune system cells.

20

CROSSING THE VALLEY OF DEATH

Despite a large number of vitiligo patients and the associated costs to society and national economies, vitiligo has traditionally not been considered a particularly attractive target for drug development. Even if it were, this wouldn't guarantee a cure.

In its ideal form, drug development is simple and elegant: take a promising idea through a series of objective experiments, register the positive outcome with the governing body, then send the cure to pharmacies worldwide. But the reality is very different.

On the one hand, less than a third of the approximate 30,000 diseases, syndromes and conditions known to mankind are treated effectively. On the other hand, the latest release of the Canadian Drug Bank database contains over 10,500 drug entries, including:

- 1,737 approved small molecule drugs,
- 870 approved biotech drugs,
- 103 nutraceuticals, and
- over 5,000 experimental drugs.

Additionally,

- 4,772 drug target-enzyme-carrier sequences are linked to these drug entries.[55]

An average drug development program costs approximately $2.6 billion.[56] Some critics suggest the true cost is closer to $150 million,[57] but others raise the bar to $5 billion.[58] Any number is big and almost unfathomable. To make your own conclusions, feel free to download this Excel chart[59] developed by Bruce Booth – an early stage venture capitalist, writer, researcher – and play with the numbers yourself.

Only one in 10,000 new compounds will be approved by the U.S. Federal Drug Administration (FDA) – after 12 or so years of research, clinical trials and doing all the paperwork. Less than one in 10 will then make enough profit to justify the investment; and an 8% figure is the consensus on drug success rate.[60] No wonder, then, that Big Pharma is reluctant to invest a huge amount into *de novo* drug development programs.

Rather, it often leaves academic researchers and biotech companies to go through the 'Valley of Death', as it's called in the industry, on their own. This term describes the period of transition when a technology under development is deemed promising, but too new to attract funding or investors.

21

DRUG MONEY TRAIL

I n the initial stages of a new drug's life cycle, research is usually funded by a university or government agency. This stage is relatively inexpensive. But, as the drug candidate works its way through the life cycle towards a more mature level, costs grow exponentially. Without sufficient funding, brave researchers risk venturing too far into the Valley of Death.

At that stage, it is no longer the university or government that determines if the product is going to move forward. A handful of executives at a pharmaceutical company would determine if the product has any future. They would determine the costs associated with bringing the product to market versus projected revenues. Revenue predictions are based on projected demand, which in turn, is based on the anticipated number of repeat sales and potential for health insurance coverage.

However, the health insurance industry isn't happy about Big Pharma's approach to the pricing of new and specialty drugs.[61] One of the terrifying things about the drug market is that competition often doesn't result in lower prices. Through an opaque and confusing system of deductibles, premiums and cost-sharing options, these costs are then extracted from consumers' pockets.

Finally, potential consumers – vitiligo patients like you and me – are being scrutinized for their willingness to pay for future treatments. Willingness-to-pay research study data from Germany indicates that annual amount for 'vitiligo healing' was $8,389 (€7,359) back in 2009.[62] This data correlates with the results of an online study more recently conducted by VR Foundation about the actual cost of vitiligo treatments and camouflage to date.[63] Further, it correlates with an assessment of the annual cost of in-clinic phototherapy sessions for vitiligo in the U.S., and national reimbursement rates by Medicare.

To date, capital has not yet flowed in a meaningful way into academic labs or biotech companies focusing on neglected diseases. The Valley of Death has become an uncrossable canyon for many vitiligo folk. But some of them have found a tiny oasis in the middle of it.

22

NON-HUMAN ANIMAL MODELS

A dilemma faced by researchers is how to prove the efficacy of scientifically promising drug candidates. FDA requires new medicines and treatments to be evaluated in a living organism before being given to humans. Cell cultures and computer simulations cannot yet emulate the complicated and sometimes unpredictable processes of a living system. For obvious ethical and safety reasons, the research cannot be performed in humans. Instead, various non-human animal, fungal, bacterial, and plant species are used as model organisms for their studies.

Of the 106 Nobel Prizes awarded for Physiology or Medicine, 94 were directly dependent on research using animals – from the very first one in 1901 until the most recent in 2017.[64]

Although predictive for many diseases, animals have proven to be poor models for human skin disease research.[65] The difficulties result from the metabolic, anatomic, and cellular differences between humans and other creatures – but the problems go even deeper than that. The further away from the human species the animal studies get, the less predictive the model will be.

Mice are commonly used as a model for studying human biology and diseases, and also as test subjects for the development of drugs. In the lab, scientists aim to produce and study the equivalent of vitiligo or other disease in mice. They often create a 'knockout' mice by turning off one of its genes, in order to see what effect this has on the animal and the disease development. For example, the mouse model used by Prof. Harris at his lab at University of Massachusetts has revealed a lot about vitiligo that has been later confirmed in humans.

Several other non-human animal models of vitiligo exist – including chicken, horse, dog, swine and even water buffalo – although the exact relevance of such models to the equivalent human vitiligo remains unclear.[66,67,68]

PART VI

THE PUBLISHING DILEMMA

~

23

THE OASIS IS SHRINKING

D rug discovery often begins in academic research labs, and the process of translating a lab discovery into a drug is fraught with difficulty. There is a tremendous gap between the time of the original discovery and getting to market.

For almost any kind of research project, scientists need money: to buy lab equipment and supplies, to run experiments, to analyze data, to pay their assistants and even themselves. What's more, access to scientific publications and libraries may cost anything from $20 per paper to $20,000 for an annual subscription. The scientific publishing business model is a truly puzzling thing, with margins higher than those of high-tech giants like Apple, Google and Amazon.[69]

THIS EXPLAINS the enormous popularity of the controversial Sci-Hub online service, which offers completely free access to pretty much any academic journal article ever published.[70] Its founder belongs to a radical wing of the open access movement. Alexandra Elbakyan, a neuroscientist from Kazakhstan, created it in 2011 to openly share knowledge with those unable to pay hefty fees. Users can simply paste a web link into a Google-like form and get instant, full access to any of the 62 million papers locked behind a paywall.

Unsurprisingly, major publishers are trying very hard to shut the website down, but it remains outside the jurisdictional reach of the U.S. courts. In support of Sci-Hub, a group of researchers and artists created a website with an open letter that likens a juggernaut scientific journal publisher to the greedy businessman in Antoine de Saint-Exupéry's *The Little Prince*.[71]

Sci-Hub is not the only way to get free access to academic papers, however. Researchers and scholars often use the hashtag #ICanHazPDF on Twitter[72] to ask fellow colleagues for paywalled articles.[73]

In bioscience, the initial grant can be around $150,000 for pilot research. Even small investments may pay off handsomely in the end. Universities can receive millions of dollars in royalties if a product from their lab is developed. But research is getting more expensive, and academic researchers cannot rely on university funding alone to pay for these expenses. Instead, they have to seek outside grants that are in increasingly short supply.

John Harris once shared a sad observation with me: "Over 40% of my time goes to writing grant proposals. Imagine how much more we could have accomplished in my lab if I could spend this time doing research?"

24

PROTECT THE SOURCE

However, scientists aren't just griping about money. To increase the chances of getting grants, scientists need published work – lots and lots of it. In turn, this encourages them to pick low risk projects, to routinely cut corners, to suppress challenging observations, to overhype their work and even to bias their research towards specific outcomes.

Grants also usually expire after two to three years, which pushes scientists away from long-term projects. Yet truly novel research takes many years longer to produce and publish results, and it doesn't always pay off.

When funds are not available in their field of interest, scientists turn to the biopharma industry. A vast majority of clinical trials are funded by either drug or medical equipment makers, which creates significant conflicts of interest. Scientists often feel compelled to keep funding sources happy and to publish safe, quick turnaround papers in order to maintain their jobs and careers.

Psst... frankly speaking, you could get almost any result you want, depending on how you set up the study – but that's another story.

Sometimes, scientists and university hospitals have financial relationships with drug and medical device manufacturing companies. Open Payments is the transparency program run by the U.S. government that collects and makes this information publicly available to help patients make informed decisions.[74]

As a result, as much as 30% of the most influential, original medical research papers later turn out to be wrong, exaggerated or are impossible to reproduce.[75] Thankfully, someone at the federal government was clearly disappointed with this colossal waste of taxpayers' money. Under new government rules, researchers will have to reveal the results of most clinical trials, including some for drugs and devices that never reach the market.[76]

However, science is still better than snake oil cures!

25

PREDATORS AND THEIR PREY

The size, wealth and influence of the scientific publishing sector is quite staggering. It weighs in somewhere between the recording and film industries in size, but is far more profitable.

Editors of top journals now have the power to not only shape a scientist's career, but the direction of science itself. Researchers understand that their chances of getting a good job, project or funding depend on getting publications into CNS – an acronym that groups together the three most prestigious journals in life sciences: *Cell*, *Nature* and *Science*. A 'reasonable' scientist nowadays will prefer to work on a topic that is popular with CNS editors, and thus likely to yield regular publications, rather than drive discoveries.

Those researchers rejected by top journals are often embraced by predatory publishers masquerading as 'open-access' journals, who charge an upfront fee to make research public but turn out to be fraudulent, without any academic credence. The shiny looks of these publishers have deceived thousands of young and inexperienced researchers, costing them millions of dollars and, for many, their reputations.

Academic science is plagued with another problem: a publication bias. Studies with positive results touting the success of a new drug or device, or those with dramatic conclusions, are far more likely to be published than negative ones. So, we only see the bright tip of the iceberg, while the bottom part with negative animal findings or failed human results remains hidden.

Science journalism is similarly full of exaggerated, conflicting, or outright misleading claims. For both universities and scientists, media attention can boost reputation and generate more funding. But research shows that science is hyped even before it reaches newsrooms.[77] Around a third of press releases from universities and non-profit research foundations were found to contain grossly exaggerated statements. Next, overstretched and overworked journalists often don't read the original research paper, instead commenting on the inflated press release, with excess optimism and an inadequate sense of limits.

When doctors want to make sense of this convoluted scientific and medical literature, they turn to the meta-analyses and systematic reviews. For many years, these were considered the gold standard for evidence, but things got completely out of hand recently.

The production of systematic reviews and meta-analyses of low quality has reached epidemic proportions. Too many meta-analyses are being generated by the scientists willing to cherry-pick facts to build narratives that suit their purpose. And that defeats one of the main purposes of these studies: to get a quick take on what really works and what doesn't. By the conservative estimate of Prof. Ioannidis, "only three percent of all meta-analyses are decent and clinically useful."[78]

TREATMENTS

PART VII

CONSIDER ALL ODDS

~

26

EMOJI AS SKIN PHOTOTYPES

D id you know the omnipresent, colorful Emoji characters in your mobile phone app are actual representations of different skin phototypes?

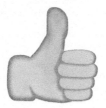

The Fitzpatrick Skin Type is a skin classification system[79] that includes six different skin types and colors in respect to their toleration to the sun:

• Type I. Pale white skin; red or blond hair; blue eyes; freckles. Common in Northern Europe and Britain. Always burns, never tans.

• Type II. White or fair skin; red or blond hair; blue, hazel, or green eyes. Common in Europe and Scandinavia. Usually burns, tans with difficulty.

- Type III. Cream white or fair skin; any eye or hair color. Common in Central and Southern Europe. Gradually tans, sometimes has a mild burn.
- Type IV. Light brown skin. Common in Asia, the Mediterranean, Latin America. Tans with ease, rarely burns.
- Type V. Dark brown skin. Common in East India, Africa, and among Native Americans. Tans very easily, rarely burns.
- Type VI. Deeply pigmented dark brown. Common in Africa and among Aboriginals. Tans very easily, very rarely burns.

This system is the standard system used by aestheticians, cosmetologists and dermatologists in order to determine how someone will respond to treatments.

As an example, a patient with Fitzpatrick skin type II will have a greater tendency toward irritation, but less for repigmentation. Individuals with skin type III are conducive to a range of treatments with minor side effects. Accordingly, the Fitzpatrick skin type VI will not be as easily irritated and will have an inordinately high tendency toward repigmentation.

27

DECODING MEDICAL JARGON

"NSV, w/o fam hist, FitzIII, Koebner, leucotr, >20% BSA. BX unremarkabl. Reccd: NB-UVB w/TCS BID, 2/w 12 wks" reads the dermatologist note brought to me by a perplexed vitiligo patient.

Huh?? Translated (and it took me a while to decipher the handwriting, as well) the note says this: "Non-segmental vitiligo, without family history of the disease, Fitzpatrick skin type III, lesions caused by skin damage, white hairs within lesions that cover more than 20% of the body surface area, biopsy normal. Recommended narrowband phototherapy with topical corticosteroids twice daily, two times per week, for 12 weeks." More understandable, but the potential for misunderstanding is still enormous.

The fact is that many patients are rightfully baffled by medical jargon, but are too embarrassed to seek clarification. Language and cultural barriers add stress to the confusion. Most of us simply pretend they understand what the doctor is saying and nod at random moments, as if in agreement.

Doctors often do not even realize they are speaking and writing in a language that no one outside the profession understands. They assume that patients will somehow navigate unfamiliar territory through this cryptic form of communication.

Yet there is an awful lot to understand. Steroids, ultraviolet radiations, lasers, calcineurin inhibitors, topical and systemic immunomodulators are among the treatments commonly prescribed for vitiligo. Then there are surgical procedures like autologous suction blister, split-thickness, punch smash and single follicular unit grafting, cultured epidermal suspensions and autologous melanocyte culture grafting. Then you have JAK inhibitors, 5-fluorouracil, prostaglandin E2, pseudocatalase, dermabrasion, vitamins, climatotherapy, and ethno-pharmacological and other adjuvant therapies. Depigmentation may also be offered, usually as a last resort (but is it really?).

My POINT IS that how does someone with little medical knowledge make an educated choice with so many treatment options, each fraught with unpredictable outcomes? So let's get down-to-earth to make sure you walk away from this book with a clear understanding of your best treatment options and their potential outcomes.

TIP: You don't have to pretend that you understand your doctor. Ask for a layman's summary in simple language. Be assertive, but friendly.

28

AN INCONVENIENT TRUTH

"How can I be brutally honest without de-motivating the very folks I am trying to nurture?" I ask myself this question before every meeting with a patient support group or a class with medical students.

The problem is that there's currently neither a cure for vitiligo, nor a universally accepted method for limiting the spread of the disease. Although many treatments are being used for its management, none are licensed specifically for vitiligo, in the EU or the U.S. (except for one, see Part Eleven, *Depigmentation Agents.*) Every vitiligo therapy used by doctors is 'off-label' – meaning it's only approved for use in *other* conditions, such as psoriasis or atopic dermatitis.

Professor Witton and colleagues analyzed 96 studies of different vitiligo treatments.[80] These studies create a foundation for treatment guidelines used by clinicians to treat patients. But they found the quality of these studies was "poor to moderate, at best." The majority of them had fewer than 50 participants and very few studies included children or segmental forms of vitiligo. The best evidence showed "short-term benefit from topical corticosteroids" and "various forms of ultraviolet radiation combined with topical preparations."

UNFORTUNATELY, this is only part of the bad news. With the available treatment options, skin color is almost never fully restored. In most of the studies done so far, repigmentation of just over 75% is considered a positive outcome. Acquired color may be a couple of shades off, either lighter or darker than normal skin tone, but tends to even out over several months. About a quarter of patients never respond to *any* treatment. In a few cases this is due to breaks in treatment protocol, while some stubborn patches simply defy explanation.

And it quickly gets pricey. Medicare in the US covers the annual cost of regular phototherapy up to $16,461 at the time of writing, but it does not cover lab tests or doctor visits, which can add thousands to the bill. In our own VRF study, 13% of those surveyed had paid more than $20,000 for treatments out of their own pocket to date.

Even after successful treatment, generalized vitiligo is likely to stage a comeback within four years. Sometimes it re-appears while patients are still busy treating other patches. Sometimes it goes into remission for the duration of the treatment and flares back right after you stop it. This is typical for many so-called 'natural remedies,' which are actually slowly intoxicating your body while keeping vitiligo at bay.

TIP: PLEASE AVOID 'NATURAL REMEDIES' sold specifically for vitiligo – less than perfect color match is a minor concern compared to the potential side effects.

29

TO TREAT OR NOT TO TREAT?

A diagnosis of vitiligo brings about many emotions because of the uncertainty it causes. *Why me? Is it treatable? Is treatment worse than the disease itself?* Even selecting the best treatment can be fraught with uncertainty, too. *How long will it take? Can I afford it? Should I try to restore my color, or erase every sign of what's left?*

Though it is not always easy, or even possible, to treat vitiligo, there is much to be gained by clearly understanding the diagnosis, the future implications of the disease, and the treatment alternatives and their side effects.

And because vitiligo affects more quality of life rather than actual lifespan, the choice between treatment and no treatment at all becomes apparent. There are many subtle nuances that can tip the scale in favor of a *Yes* or *No* answer, or freeze it in the middle.

Factors to consider include age of patient and disease onset, type of vitiligo and localization, familial and disease history, overall health condition and comorbidities, living and working environments, prospects of frequent travel or military service, financial situation, access to certain treatments, and most importantly – personal motivation.

Many have dealt with vitiligo while remaining in the public eye, maintaining a positive outlook, and having a successful career. Winnie Harlow has become a top fashion model while celebrating her skin as it is. In contrast, model Breanne Rice successfully hid her vitiligo during 10 years in the fashion industry, before moving on to become a nutritionist. Lee Thomas found a therapy that worked for him halfway across the world, while partially covering his spots as a morning TV show anchor in Detroit.

A long list of famous vitiligans features elected officials, businessmen, athletes, actors, radio and TV hosts in almost every country.[81] However, for every successful life story there are thousands of untold tales of discrimination and bullying.

FOR CHILDREN and teens with vitiligo, my answer would be *Yes*. They respond better to treatments, have a daily routine that can include home-based therapy, and they will thank parents for this when they grow up.

For adults, the answer is not so obvious. A dark-skinned patient with an early stage disease is a solid candidate for treatment. Late stage disease may present a challenge, even for a vitiligo specialist.

Fair-skinned patients should be warned by a dermatologist of an expected weak response to treatments. They are best-advised to seek effective cosmetic camouflage and sunscreen for lesions on exposed skin.

'Active surveillance' – where one carefully monitors stable, minor vitiligo patches via periodic checkups – could be an acceptable alternative for those not yet decided. Unwarranted treatments may exhaust the patient, and lead to side effects including ones unrelated to skin.

NOTE: It takes unwavering determination, strict adherence to protocol, time and money to treat vitiligo and keep it from coming back.

30

ACTIVITY, LOCATION, TIME AND COMPLIANCE

W hile it is not possible to predict what will work best for which patients, there are four variables that can help us make an educated guess about treatment course and outcomes. These variables work somewhat differently for segmental and non-segmental vitiligo, so be sure to talk to a vitiligo specialist before any further thought.

Disease activity is the first variable to consider. Lesions that are new, or have expanded within the last year, indicate 'active' vitiligo, which responds poorly to re-pigmentation treatments – especially micro-surgery. In this case, therapy should first be focused on halting the disease, rather than repigmentation (we will get later to this in Part Nine. *Restoring Pigmentation.*)

Lesion location on the skin is the second variable, which also defines the likelihood of successful treatment. This largely depends on the number of hair follicles present in the skin (as we've seen in chapter *Elusive Melanocytes*). Areas of the skin with large numbers of hairs have a good chance of recovery. Best results are often reported on the face and neck.

On the flip side, sites with little hair – such as hands, wrists, feet, ankles, knees and elbows – have a poor chance of repigmentation. If there are dark hairs within the white spot, there is a good chance of recovery, but if the hairs have turned white, the outlook is poorer.

Our third variable is time. Childhood vitiligo has a better treatment prognosis. Early treatment – ideally within three months of a lesion first appearing – delivers faster, better and longer-lasting results. As a rule of thumb, spots that develop more slowly are also more likely to be successfully treated, compared to those spreading fast. Signs of quick skin response to therapy and dotted repigmentation – typically within the first month – raise the chances for quicker skin color restoration.

Lastly, we come to compliance. Positive treatment results stem from strict compliance to the protocol, typically within one year. Extensive travel, or an extra busy work or school schedule can obviously get in the way, but this lowers the chances of a positive treatment outcome.

PART VIII

TREATMENT TOOLS

31

VITILIGO SCORE

I was enjoying the *Nutcracker* ballet at the Bolshoi Theater, Moscow when my five-year-old son asked a funny question "Why is that mad man in the orchestra swinging around when nobody is looking at him?" The mad man in question was the conductor, who was creating an inspiring atmosphere for the audience on that Christmas Eve.

Of course, any decent professional orchestra can play a classic symphony with their eyes shut. But it takes a good conductor to bring it into sync with the tempo of the prima ballerina on the stage. The conductor also keeps the musicians' spirit and energy up during a long and demanding performance.

Treating vitiligo is similar to staging a ballet performance, with its delicate balance of music and action. While you can self-prescribe and self-medicate vitiligo, there's a high chance you will miss a start, skip a few notes, go at the wrong tempo or even be wildly out of sync with the rest of your body. You need your own conductor – a skin specialist – to keep it all in order.

In order to impress spectators with the flawless tone of your skin, consider medications as notes and your doctor's prescription as a musical score. They must go together exactly as prescribed, without missing a beat.

Certain medications lend themselves easily to personification as instruments. Just like a symphonic orchestra isn't whole without the strings, woodwinds, brass and percussion, vitiligo treatment wouldn't be complete without a kind of phototherapy, topical creams, internal medications and supplements.

Phototherapy is your principal instrument for the duration of the act, usually slowing tempo down towards the end of the performance. Creams and medications play loudly at certain points, depending on what's happening on the stage that is your skin and body. Supplements determine the mood and energy of the act.

A good doctor will intervene like an experienced conductor, exactly when needed. Without speaking too much, your doc can adjust certain instruments so they play a perfect tune together.

Continuing with our musical analogy, the choice of main instruments depends on the dancers – the spots – on our improvised vitiligo stage, and the complex interactions between them throughout the play.

We should already know what kind of vitiligo act is unfolding before our eyes as (I hope!) you will have talked to a dermatologist by now. And while the act is, by nature, totally unpredictable, we can make an educated guess of its future direction based on the number of dancers, their activity and location:

A SINGLE STUBBORN dancer anywhere on the stage may require some surgical instruments to remove it for good. The same goes for small groups hanging on one side of the stage only.

A SLOW-MO ACT – a few erratic dancers on the backstage – can unfold over years. This would require a combination of topical therapies and a type of light treatment, possibly as simple as sunlight.

A MODERATE ACTIVITY of some of the dancers in the mid-stage can go either way – into a slow-mo or high energy act, and thus would require additional medications to keep it under reasonable control.

A DRAMA-LIKE ACTIVITY of groups of dancers can quickly spread like wildfire and involve everyone on the stage. Bigger instruments need to come in here, depending on the complexity of interactions between actors.

DESPITE THEIR APPEAL, 'ALTERNATIVE MEDICINES' are rarely instruments on their own. They lack specific tune and thus can only be used as an ambient music that puts an emphasis on the atmosphere over structured melody. Now as we have figured out what's going on and where it's heading, we can take a closer look at our instruments and ready them for use.

32

LIGHTS UP!

L ight therapy, also known as phototherapy in a narrow sense, has long been considered the 'gold standard' of vitiligo treatment. Intense light of a certain wavelength produces biological reactions within the skin that lead to clearing of lesions.

Phototherapy is a relatively safe and effective non-drug treatment option. It is good for kids and seniors, pregnant or lactating women, and those with certain health conditions. Treatment can be applied to the whole body or it can be precisely focused on affected areas to minimize exposure of uninvolved skin.

It has two modes of action in helping to combat vitiligo. Firstly, intense light stimulates activity of melanocytes – cells that produce pigment in the skin. Secondly, light halts the destruction of melanocytes by the immune system, which erroneously identifies them as intruders.

Sunlight, ultraviolet lamps and lasers are the best-known phototherapy tools. And because good results require a long term commitment and some expense, I suggest we concentrate on the basics of phototherapy first. If you wish to dig deeper into the clinical aspects, I recommend a systematic review by Jung Min Bae.[82] (If you're in a rush, feel free to skip for now and go straight to the chapter *Narrowband UVB*.)

33

ABC'S OF UV

U ltraviolet (UV) light is the part of sunlight that reaches the surface of Earth in abundance. This narrow strip of the broad spectrum of sunlight is further divided into three types:

UV-A: 320 to 400 nanometers
UV-B: 290 to 320 nanometers
UV-C: 100 to 290 nanometers

When UV and visible radiation reach the skin, one part is reflected, and the other part is absorbed into the various skin layers, which all respond differently:

- UVA are rays that *age*. They are able to penetrate deep into the dermis – the second layer of the skin – and cause damage that contributes to oxidative stress and cancers of the skin.
- UVB are the rays that *burn*. They penetrate only the outermost layer of the skin – the epidermis. There,

photons are mainly absorbed by cell components like proteins or DNA.

- UVC are the rays that cause *no harm*. They are almost completely absorbed by the ozone layer and the little that does reach the skin has no effect.

34

PUVA: PHOTOCHEMOTHERAPY

The first phototherapeutic device for vitiligo treatment, introduced back in the late 1970s, was the UVA light. This name is given to the waveband of sunlight ranging from 320 nm to 400 nm.

It is either used alone and known as 'broadband UVA' or in combination with psoralens that sensitize your skin to sunlight and known as 'PUVA,' or photochemotherapy. Although moderately effective for clearing a variety of skin diseases, PUVA's limitations and adverse side effects have led to a decline in usage in recent years.[83] Nonetheless, PUVA is still used in many countries in Central Europe, Central and South America, and Africa, so we should look at its proper use and limitations.

PUVA THERAPY CONSISTS of the skin application or oral intake of psoralen followed by exposure to UVA light. Psoralens are compounds found in many plants, which make the skin temporarily sensitive to UVA. Medicine psoralens include methoxsalen and trisoralen – the latter is slightly safer than the former.

For oral PUVA, psoralen capsules are taken two hours before a treatment appointment. For topical PUVA, psoralen lotions are applied to the skin 10-20 minutes before treatment. For bathwater PUVA, the patient soaks in a bath containing a solution of psoralens for half-an-hour prior to the procedure.

PUVA treatments are performed two to three times a week, on non-consecutive days. During the procedure, the patient stands either inside a tall booth that wraps around the body, or in front of panels with six-foot long fluorescent bulbs that illuminate one side of the body at a time. The patient is usually dressed only in underpants for whole body exposure, wearing dark goggles to protect the eyes from exposure to UV radiation during the procedure.

If vitiligo affects hands or feet only, the patient may be directed towards a smaller unit. However, these devices are usually ineffective for extremities and thus should be re-considered with your doctor.

Exposure time and UVA radiation dose will be gradually increased from one minute up to half-an-hour. Shortly after the treatment, a mild skin reaction develops, which turns white lesions pink for several hours and then fades away under normal conditions. This effect is called *erythema*. It is a necessary, although unsightly, part of treatment in order to deliver an adequate dose and clear white spots.

A trained specialist should find the fine balance between a biologically effective dose and potential consequences of the UV radiation exposure. In practice, however, doctors and nurses working with UV equipment tend to overexpose patients from the very beginning. A burn often happens 48 to 72 hours after the first two or three treatments, especially in light-skinned people. Treatment time and dose must be adjusted accordingly,[84] and one or more treatments should be skipped.

Most patients will see a significant improvement in face and upper body in four to six months of twice-weekly treatments, but they should continue for up to two years to achieve a long-lasting effect. Results for hands and feet are less encouraging. Complete repigmentation cannot be guaranteed and relapse is possible after a few months or years.

Where PUVA cabinets are unavailable, dermatologists may recommend exposing skin to sunlight after taking psoralens. Unfortunately, sunlight is unpredictable so it is difficult to get the correct dose. Too little, and it is ineffective. Too much, and it burns the skin. Sunlight is not suitable for therapy in most of Northern Europe or Northern USA, but is adequate in Africa, Asia, and the Middle East during certain periods of the day.

PUVA THERAPY HAS ITS LIMITATIONS, safety concerns and adverse side effects due to both UV radiation and psoralen properties. The most common short-term side effects are erythema, pruritus, xerosis and phototoxic reactions. Temporary mild pricking or itching of the skin is common after treatment, and skin often feels dry, which may be addressed with anti-histamine tablets and moisturizers. Nausea occurs in a quarter of those treated with psoralens, but this can be minimized by taking them with food and antiemetic tablets.

Long-term PUVA side effects include premature skin aging, discoloration, wrinkles, broken blood vessels, gastric and ocular damage, and an increased risk of skin cancer. Because of psoralen's toxicity, PUVA therapy can be performed only in adults, and should be avoided during pregnancy. Patients are strongly advised to avoid sunbathing, perfumed cosmetics and applications of coal tar for one day after each PUVA session.

NOTE: PUVA can cause cataracts in the unprotected eyes. Patients must wear protective goggles both during and after the procedure. Put on wrap-around sunglasses with UVA protection for 24 hours following PUVA treatment – even indoors, if any sunlight comes into the room.

NARROWBAND UVB

N arrowband UVB (NB-UVB) phototherapy is the treatment of choice for many skin conditions today. It was first used to treat vitiligo in 1997, but twenty years later it is still an unaffordable luxury for patients in many countries.

'Narrowband' refers to specific waveband of UV radiation, stretching from 308 nm to 312 nm. This range is believed to be the most beneficial component of natural sunlight for vitiligo. From the patient's perspective, PUVA and NB-UVB are very similar in appearance, but this is deceptive. There are more differences than similarities between them, in both therapeutic mechanism and outcomes.

Research data supports the practical observations that NB-UVB produces better repigmentation than PUVA, with better color match and fewer side effects.[85,86] NB-UVB therapy is also better tolerated, and could be used on expecting or nursing women, and children.

Getting The Right UVB Dose

At your first day at the doctor's office you may have to go through a light test before treatment begins. An individual skin response to UVB depends on its Fitzpatrick type, daily exposure and sensitivity to sunlight. Doctor can try different doses of UVB on small areas of your skin – about 1 cm each – to calculate your safe starting dose. The next day, some of these areas will develop a sunburn-like redness, while the color of others will remain unchanged. The lowest dose necessary to produce just perceptible redness is known as MED, or the Minimal Erythemal Dose.

This test maybe inconvenient for doctors and difficult to perform accurately in some clinics. Instead, it can be reasonably assumed that prominent vitiligo lesions will have Fitzgerald skin type I, which has MED of 400 millijoules per square centimeter (mJ/cm²). These clinics will use pre-defined dose increase schedules, instead of the light test.

A commonly used NB-UVB treatment protocol suggests the first exposure to NB-UVB at 70% of MED, followed by a 20% dose increase on a weekly basis to a maximum allowed dose. Other doctors may start phototherapy based on how each person recalls their skin's reaction to sun exposure.

A slight pink cast over white lesions, which begins two to six hours after exposure, peaks at 12-18 hours after exposure and fades within 48 hours, is thought to be an optimal response to UV therapy.[87]

Managing Over and Under-Dose

After short exposure on the first visit, subsequent visits will feature increasing amounts of UVB. Unfortunately, all too frequently patients are burned during their first two weeks of treatments.

Here's how a nurse might deal with the most common situations during the course of phototherapy:

- White lesions, no color change: follow protocol and increase dose by 10% from the previous session.
- Light pink lesions (erythema without discomfort): maintain the dose without skipping the treatment.
- Pink lesions (erythema with some discomfort): omit one session and then repeat previous dose.
- Red lesions (sore erythema but without swelling): pause until settled, reduce subsequent treatment by 10%. Emollients and analgesia should be offered.
- Marked pain, severe erythema or blistering: hold off further treatment until if fades, then reduce by 25%. In the meantime, review alternatives with your doctor.

Skipped treatments require dosage adjustment depending on the number of calendar days missed.[88] If you missed less than a week, the dose may still be minimally increased. After an eight to 11-day break, hold the dose constant. 12-20 missed days will result in a dose decrease by 25%, and by 50% for another 21-27 days. You should be starting over from MED after 28+ days of interruption.

UVB Treatment Duration

Study after study confirms that the earlier the patient is treated, the better the response, especially for lesions on the face, neck and trunk.[89,90] Ideally, vitiligo should be treated within three months of it first appearing because as the condition progresses, it becomes harder – although no means impossible – to treat. Even 10, 20 or 30-year old vitiligo spots may be re-pigmented with enough patience using a combination of narrowband UVB with other therapies.

Most patients will notice some results after 24-36 thrice-weekly treatments, but sometimes it takes three to four months before any repigmentation is seen. The initial duration will be measured in seconds rather than minutes, and gradually increased by 5-20% with every session, until it reaches just the right level for your skin.

Signs of *some* repigmentation are observed in the majority of adult patients with non-segmental vitiligo, although *complete* repigmentation is only found in a minority. In an open study by Prof. Westerhof, after eight months of phototherapy treatment, less than half of patients showed a 'marked' response, while others showed a 'moderate' or 'mild' response.[91]

In children, vitiligo stops progressing after 12 weeks of NB-UVB treatments, while repigmentation is commonly achieved by the end of the first year of treatments.[92] An average 34 treatment visits are required to achieve 50% repigmentation. Prof. Silverberg suggests starting twice-weekly phototherapy after the age of five, as younger children have difficulty standing still during the procedure.[93]

No consensus exists as to the *optimum duration* of phototherapy, and practice varies widely. Prof. Harris from mild-weathered Boston recommends NB-UVB treatment to be performed thrice-weekly for the first three months, and twice-weekly thereafter.[94]

Prof. Andrija Stanimirovic from sun-kissed Croatia, suggests scheduled sunbathing from June to September, then NB-UVB thrice-weekly for the rest of the year. In a case of fast-spreading vitiligo, he begins with thrice-weekly NB-UVB for 24 weeks, or recommends the Dead Sea climatotherapy for three to four weeks.

There are currently no recommendations for a *maximum number* of treatments. Fitzpatrick skin types I and II are known to repigment weaker compared to types III and IV, regardless of the number of phototherapy sessions, and are prone to quick relapse. A limit on the number of treatments for these skin types was arbitrarily set at 200 treatments. Most adult patients with extensive vitiligo and darker skin types – Fitzpatrick type III-IV – would require between 180 and 220 sessions over a period of one-

and-a-half to two years to achieve a near complete repigmentation.

NB-UVB sessions may be stopped if no repigmentation occurs after the first three months of no-skip treatment, or in case of unsatisfactory response (less than 25% color restoration) after six months of treatment.

TIP: Keep records documenting each treatment including date, exposure time and degree of erythema. Any withheld treatments should be recorded with explanations. Take photos of your lesions on the first day of every month to monitor progress, response to treatments and safety.

36

TARGETED PHOTOTHERAPY

Targeted phototherapy, produced by focused lights, is a newer form of NB-UVB phototherapy, with both advantages and disadvantages. You may encounter devices with different technologies, such as excimer laser (308 nm), intense pulse light systems (304-308 nm), non-laser light sources (290-310 nm) and micro-focused systems (300-320 nm).

Lasers may seem magical due to their unique properties of micro-focusing, high-intensity, ultrashort pulses and all that marketing stuff. But a laser is just an expensive light bulb and its radiation follows the same rules as radiation from an NB-UVB tube. Whether the light used to stimulate melanocyte growth was generated by a laser, or a filtered incandescent lamp of the same wavelength, makes no difference to results.

In a recent meta-review Mysore and colleagues argue that all forms of targeted phototherapy are useful in vitiligo, but there is no evidence that they are vastly superior to traditional phototherapy.[95] Excimer laser may produce faster repigmentation than NB-UVB in early stages of treatment, but in the long run they both have similar efficacy.[96] And because these devices use a similar

mechanism to NB-UVB, the same basic precautions and warn-
ings should apply.

The main benefits of targeted phototherapy are the safety and
ease of administration. Once-weekly treatment is acceptable and
effective, compared to twice or thrice-weekly requirement for NB-
UVB sessions. Also, because the light is tightly focused on a small
area, unaffected skin is spared from irradiation and hence from
unwanted hyperpigmentation and photoaging.[97,98,99] The maneu-
verable laser head allows treatment of difficult areas such as the
scalp, nose, genitals, oral mucosa and ears. And a small hand-
piece looks less scary to children, who often feel intimidated by a
6-ft tall UVB booth.

But a strength can also be a weakness, and focused light is not
good for treating large skin areas. For the average vitiligo patient
– with seven white patches covering nearly 15% of the body, or
2.58 ft² (0.24 m²) in total – focused light is not feasible, as it takes
too long to treat this extensive area with laser dots, and it will
quickly become prohibitively expensive.

37

HOME-BASED PHOTOTHERAPY

Home therapy with NB-UVB lamps may be a great alternative for many vitiligo patients.[100] Home-based and clinic-based therapies have similar outcomes and safety profiles, but home phototherapy is more cost-effective.[101,102] Eligibility, protocols and precautions are essentially the same as discussed above, with one important addition: it should be supervised by an experienced doctor.

The benefits of home-based phototherapy speak for themselves:

- An effective, drug-free treatment.
- Easy to operate in the privacy of your home.
- No travel needed, which saves a lot of time and money.
- Much easier to keep to a treatment schedule.
- New devices have built-in software, so doctors can control dosage remotely and monitor compliance.
- In Canada and the USA, device purchase is covered by many health insurance plans or can be deducted from your taxes as a medical expense tax credit.

Home phototherapy has been used in Europe since 1979. In some parts of Scotland there is even a UVB phototherapy service for selected and well-trained patients to use at home, with trained phototherapy nurses remotely monitoring the treatment progress.[103]

But many physicians remain unaware of the benefits of home phototherapy. American professors Lim and Lebwohl even issued a collective 'call for action' for proper training of physicians in phototherapy.[104] However, many of those familiar with the matter still refuse to oversee home phototherapy, because of the common use of unregistered devices and potential for adverse reactions.

Home phototherapy devices range from hand-held and table-top devices for localized treatment, to freestanding or walk-in units for full body treatment. Well-known companies producing home phototherapy units include Daavlin, National Biological Corp. and UVA Biotek from the USA, Solarc Systems from Canada, or Kernel and Sigma Med from China.

Newcomers like the Californian company Clarify Medical offer portable devices with light emitting diodes (LEDs) instead of lasers or tubes. In general, they are virtually unbreakable – a bit more expensive than handheld UVB lamps, but far more convenient and safe. They have a built-in rechargeable battery, LCD screen and can even remotely communicate with your doctor through a mobile app.[105]

Regulations in the USA and Canada require a prescription for purchase of any phototherapy light systems, while in the EU and most other countries you can simply order them online and have them promptly delivered to your doorstep.[106,107]

TIP: Tanning beds in commercial salons are no substitute for UVB phototherapy for vitiligo. Their poorly calibrated lamps emit mostly ultraviolet light type A (UVA) – not therapeutic ultra-violet type B (UVB) – in unpredictable doses, which can damage the skin, cause premature skin aging and increase the risk of skin cancer.

38

CONTRA-INDICATIONS AND SIDE EFFECTS

The major contraindications for whole-body phototherapy are the use of certain medications or substances that may interfere with UVB rays and cause burning or stinging sensations in the skin.[108] These symptoms usually appear within 24 hours of the exposure and resolve within two to seven days of stopping the drug therapy.

The full list compiled by the FDA is 15-pages long and contains hundreds of generic and brand names.[109] Not everyone who uses these medications, swallowed or applied to the skin, will experience an adverse side effect from phototherapy. But if you are using any of them, you should take precautions and talk to your dermatologist.

These are a few to be aware of:

- acne medications with isotretinoin/acitretin,
- antibiotics with quinolones or tetracyclines,
- antimicrobials with sulfonamides,
- antipsychotics with phenothiazine,
- cardiac drugs with amiodarone/nifedipine/quinidine/diltiazem,

- contraceptives, oral and estrogens like birth control pills,
- diabetic drugs with sulfonylureas/glyburide, and
- painkillers with NSAID, such as naproxen or piroxicam.

Certain cosmetics and dyes, deodorants, perfumes, essential oils, and anti-bacterial soaps may cause mild skin irritation after phototherapy. A shower before the session – especially if you are on a home phototherapy regimen – will minimize potential risks. Some plants – including limes, celery, and parsley – contain compounds called furocoumarins that make some people's skin more sensitive to the effects of UV light.

Even traces of certain sunscreens that are meant to protect your skin from excessive light can cause a rash after UVB exposure. Avoid sunscreens with PABA and benzophenone ingredients in favor of those containing physical blockers, such as zinc oxide or titanium dioxide.

If you have a history of skin cancer, lupus, xeroderma, arsenic intake or previous treatment with ionizing radiation or immuno-suppressive medications, you must be evaluated by a dermatologist before prescription of UVB therapy.

Caution should be exercised by patients with Fitzpatrick skin types I and II, who tend to burn easily. They will see an increased contrast between pigmented and depigmented areas, which can be bothersome and sometimes a reason to stop phototherapy.

The most common side effects of UVB phototherapy are dry and itchy skin, redness and associated discomfort. These can be minimized with emollients, antihistamines and mild painkillers.

Prolonged UVB phototherapy may also cause premature skin aging, although it is less pronounced than after UVA therapy. The symptoms of photoaging differ from one case to another, and can include fine and coarse wrinkles, drooping skin, broken blood vessels, discoloration, or a yellowish tint and leathery texture to the skin.[110] To counter these effects, you should quit active or passive smoking, reduce consumption of sweets, and use skincare products with antioxidants like vitamins C and E, extracts of green tea or soy bean.[111]

39

FOLLOW-UP AFTER PHOTOTHERAPY

After successfully completing a phototherapy treatment, approximately half of patients may develop vitiligo lesions in repigmented skin within the first year.[112] Twice-daily application of 0.1% tacrolimus ointment is effective in preventing the depigmentation of previously treated patches.[113] Supportive, low-dose phototherapy might also be helpful for keeping vitiligo at bay, although there is no general consensus on this matter.

Ongoing follow-up by a dermatologist is recommended for patients who have received prolonged phototherapy - especially PUVA - to monitor for any signs of skin cancer.

TIP: Disclose all your skincare products, supplements and medications to your doctor before starting phototherapy. You should inform the phototherapy staff of any new medicines prescribed or purchased, including herbal preparations.

BOTTOM LINE. Phototherapy tools for non-segmental vitiligo can be used as follows:

- PUVA: not recommended, unless there are no other options.
- NB-UVB: for treatment of active, localized or extensive vitiligo, at clinic or home.
- Laser: for treatment of small lesions with low activity.

PART IX

RESTORING PIGMENTATION

~

As I noted before, vitiligo should ideally be treated within three months of its first appearance, because as the condition progresses it becomes harder – although by no means impossible – to treat. Even ten, twenty or thirty-year old vitiligo spots may be re-pigmented with enough patience.

40

ONE, TWO, THREE – GO!

The hierarchy between treatments is organized differently for different diseases, with blurred lines between regimens. In common diseases like flu the first line is drawn between over-the-counter drugs and those to be prescribed only by a health professional. On the other hand, in cancer treatments the first line is reserved for big guns that have the most effectiveness in terms of shrinking tumors and improving survival chances.

At the end of the day, it's just a nomenclature. It's not that first line treatment is too weak or too strong. First line therapy is the treatment regimen that is generally recommended for initial treatment of a certain disease, and so is judged better for you to begin with. There are some patients who get second-line and third-line treatments that are better than their first-line treatments, but this is not always the case.

First Line Treatments: Stuff on the Skin

First line for vitiligo is dotted with topical treatments — corticosteroids along with calcineurin inhibitors, which are widely available at reasonable cost.[114] These are medications that you regularly apply to your skin, with the primary aim of stopping progression and thus stabilizing the disease.

And it is not uncommon for oral medications from the second line to be used as a first response to stop fast-spreading lesions.[115]

According to the European guidelines for management of vitiligo, topical treatments have the best effect on the upper body, with dark skin, and with recent lesions.

Topical treatments have many advantages over oral medications that you ingest, as they bypass your internal organs, thereby avoiding many adverse effects. However, a topical treatment regimen requires prolonged use of these medications, which often exceeds the usual safe recommended periods for corticosteroids.[116] This may result in adverse side effects like skin atrophy, acne or other unsightly conditions. On rare occasions, patients with large treatment areas and children may also experience insomnia, agitation, weight gain, and adrenal insufficiency.

Calcineurin inhibitors — tacrolimus, and less frequently pimecrolimus — are another effective topical choice, especially for children, without the adverse effects of corticosteroids.[117] They may be used on the eyelids, face, neck and genitals – areas where steroid therapy is less desirable. The most frequent side effect of these medications is a burning sensation during the first 10–14 days of application, which is usually transient. Also, a common facial flushing after alcohol intake can be bothersome for some patients undergoing this treatment.

Many vitiligo experts tend to 'pulse' first line treatments, meaning intermittent use of corticosteroids and calcineurin inhibitors for an approximate two-week duration, usually *b.i.d.* (abbreviation of the Latin phrase *bis in die*, meaning twice a day) for six months.

Here are some of the treatment suggestions that must be

further adjusted by a dermatologist to suit a patient's situation and local drug availability:

- If an adult patient just has a few, relatively stable spots, since the mid-1970s a potent topical steroid – such as 0.1% betamethasone valerate – is commonly tried first, *b.i.d.* In modern practice, it is often alternated with tacrolimus every two weeks for six months, to minimize the risk of skin atrophy. For spots on an adult's face, eyelids, genitals, breasts or underarms a less irritating medicine like 0.1% tacrolimus, *b.i.d.*, is preferable, and 0.03% tacrolimus is reserved for the sensitive skin of kids aged 2-15 years.

- If an adult patient does not respond to the previous option, then high-potency drugs such as 0.05% clobetasol propionate can be used *b.i.d.* for up to 8 weeks, after which it should be slowly reduced to a lesser strength.[118] On sensitive areas like face, neck or groin it should be used once daily. Dr. Richard Wittal from Sydney, Australia, reports good outcomes of a pulse treatment with 0.1% clobetasol, alternating with 0.1% tacrolimus ointment in a one week on/one week off regimen.

- If a patient has rapidly expanding vitiligo, with new spots appearing every week or existing ones getting bigger, a dermatologist may suggest taking oral steroids until the disease is stabilized. At a vitiligo clinic in Zagreb, Prof. Stanimirovic prescribes adults with an oral minipulse dexamethasone 4 mg, to be taken after a meal, two days a week for 16 weeks. Children get a half dose for 12 weeks.

Although frequently prescribed, vitamin D analogs – particularly calcipotriol and tacalcitol – have failed to convince vitiligo specialists of their efficacy as a monotherapy. Nevertheless, says Prof. Silverberg, they can be used adjunctively to improve steroid treatment outcomes and reduce steroid usage. Erythema, dryness, stinging, and burning have been reported as the most common side effects of their use.

The results of the first line therapy are moderately successful. Nearly half of adult patients and three-quarters of children report vitiligo stabilization and substantial repigmentation, especially in the sun-exposed areas.

Second Line Treatments: Light and Medicines

If your dermatologist calls for a second line treatment, this does *not* mean you got the wrong treatment first time. It is just a different treatment that is likely to be effective, with a twist.

(If you jumped to this page and skipped the basics of light therapy, I urge you to read Part Eight first!)

Phototherapy is usually arranged as a second defense line, when topical treatments either stopped the advance or failed to deal with widespread vitiligo. It is often fortified with oral medicines, which makes this combination remarkably more effective than any of these treatments on their own.[119]

NB-UVB with ubiquitous 0.1% tacrolimus ointment is at the forefront of second line treatments.[120] Dr. Ramaiah use phototherapy in combination with a basic Fibroblast Growth Factor (bFGF)[120], in a topical drug form widely available in India.

Prof. Lomonosov from Moscow, Russia, begins treatments with a proven immonumodulator to quickly stop vitiligo progression,[122,123] then switches to a regular UVB protocol. As so often happens, the drug manufacturer couldn't justify the enormous expense of its official registration for vitiligo, so the drug is used 'off-label' for vitiligo and other immune-imbalanced conditions by dermatologists in Kazakhstan, Russia, Ukraine and the Baltic States.

Oral use of steroids has been sparingly reported as an emergency tool to arrest the activity of fast spreading vitiligo. Intermittent oral administration of steroids like betamethasone or dexamethasone was pioneered in India in the late 1980s.[124] Within one to three months a *progressive* disease is usually stabilized, and within four months repigmentation is observed in the majority of patients. However, they are not effective in repigmenting a *stable* vitiligo, and long-term adverse effects contraindicate their common use. The drawback is a higher relapse when reducing these medications.

In a nutshell, combination interventions are superior to monotherapies but, because there are so many options and variables to consider, you should discuss them with your dermatologist.

Third Line Treatments: Surgical Methods

Third line treatments are reserved mainly for adult patients with stable, segmental or focal vitiligo, which does not respond to other treatments, has well-defined border lesions, and has no history of Koebner response. Only a handful of patients would truly qualify for these interventions, so we'll just touch upon them lightly.

Surgical techniques are divided into two basic types: transplantation of tissues and transplantation of cells. Both techniques seem to have much the same success rate.[125] Cell transplantation is a more expensive, time-consuming procedure that requires specialized staff, but provides a near-perfect color match.

The aim is to refill depleted melanocyte reservoirs with cells from a normally pigmented donor site. An important advantage of surgical treatments is the possibility of treating large areas. Rare complications include infection, hematoma, color changes at the donor site and tissue rejection at the new site.

Complete repigmentation of *segmental* vitiligo usually takes place between 2-3 months and one year, and rarely requires follow-up procedures. Surgical treatment of a *non-segmental* vitiligo should be combined with UVB follow-up for the best outcome and long-term stability.

Vitiligo surgery has to be performed in a specialized dermatological clinic under local anesthesia. I have personally visited well-equipped and staffed clinics in Chandigarh (India), Bern (Switzerland), Boston and Detroit (USA), Shenyang (China) and Shymkent (Kazakhstan) that help desperate patients regain confidence and claim their lives back.[126]

Childhood vitiligo is rarely treated with surgery. In children, progress of the disease is difficult to predict, although they respond better to medical management than adults. Sometimes, surgery has to be carried out under general anesthesia, which bears an additional risk factor for children.

Between The Lines: an Experimental Zone

There are several experimental treatments that are showing promising results as an 'off-label' treatment for vitiligo:

- A low dose medicine approach[127] that aims to rebalance the dysregulated immune response and stimulate melanocyte production is becoming popular in Italy. Two-thirds of patients with moderate vitiligo reported considerable improvement following treatment with oral drops made by GUNA®. The low dose therapy is arguably effective in itself, and even more so when overlapped with NB-UVB treatments.[128] No side effects or contra-indications were reported.

- Topical janus kinase (JAK) inhibitors, such as ruxolitinib and tofacitinib, have a credible mechanism for improving vitiligo. In a recent study conducted at Tufts Medical Center in Boston (USA) twice-daily application of 1.5% topical ruxolitinib showed promising results in facial lesions.[129] A moderate efficacy of topical JAK inhibitors is balanced with mild side effects.

- Afamelanotide, a synthetic analog of alpha-melanocyte–stimulating hormone (α-MSH) made by Clinuvel®. A grain-sized, 10-day release skin implant is seen to moderately speed up repigmentation, when used in conjunction with regular phototherapy.[130,131] It works on facial and upper extremity lesions in dark skin types, pretty much like other treatments. Adverse reactions include nausea and abdominal pain. Hyperpigmentation of normal skin and less-than-perfect color match make afamelanotide a complicated choice.

I remain hopeful that future developments in vitiligo treatments will create effective, safe and affordable medicines - probably within the next 10-15 years. If you are interested in taking part in clinical trials of new therapies, start with the online service of the U.S. National Institutes of Health.[132]

Terra Incognita: Placenta Extracts

Placenta is a lifeline for the baby in the womb. It is loaded with an array of biological substances that possess immense therapeutic potential but, after birth, it is usually disposed of along with other medical waste.

Scientists use placenta in various research fields like cancer, genetics, immunology, reproduction, toxicology, and tissue engineering. Cuba, Brazil, India and, most notably, Israel are actively developing new products from human placenta to feed a growing trend. Though it has many therapeutic applications, and been used since as early as the 1500s, public perspectives of this phenomenon are unclear and health concerns are growing.[133]

Prof. Miyares from Cuba reported in 2009 the use of an ointment, consisting of 50% alcoholic extract of human placenta with added calcium chloride.[134] Applied once-daily with graded sun exposure, it led to complete repigmentation in a quarter of patients, and notable repigmentation in half of patients after more than one year of treatment. No side effects were reported, and it was deemed suitable for children, adults and elderly people. Contra-indications were very few, including age of the disease, its active phase, light Fitzpatrick skin type, and prior use of psoralens, corticosteroids or cytokines.

TIP: Don't scramble to get an experimental treatment for vitiligo like HSP70i, JAK inhibitor, prostaglandin, or simvastatin just yet. There's always a chance they will work in mice or some people, but researchers just haven't figured out exactly who that is yet.

BOTTOM LINE: In my opinion, there is still no good data-backed argument either *for* or *against* the use of placenta extracts in vitiligo therapy. Unless you have exhausted other options, my recommendation is to hold off treatment with placenta extracts for now.

41

COMPLEMENTARY MEDICINES

Y ou'll find a wide range of books on complementary medicines in every bookstore, health food outlet, and naturopath office – not to mention a vast amount of information on the internet.

Complementary medicines can largely be divided into two types:

- medical systems, such as Ayurveda, homeopathy, naturopathy, acupuncture, and

- biologic therapies, including all kinds of folk medicines, diets, vitamins, and supplements.

Complementary therapies share a core belief that illness occurs when the whole body is out of balance. But the very definition of illness is different both within and between these groups, and so are the treatment approaches and medicines.

For example, illness in Ayurveda is defined as an imbalance of the normal ratio of three *doshas*: *vata* that controls the body's nervous system and movement, *pitta* that controls digestion and metabolism, and *kapha* that is responsible for lubrication and strength. Ayurvedic treatment follows the principle that opposites balance and so cure each other, which is in stark contrast to the homeopathic *Law of Similars*.

Traditional Chinese medicine, meanwhile, views illness as a disruption of the dynamic force called Qi, which flows across the body through a mesh of invisible channels, or meridians. Any pathology creates a congestion of forces in certain areas and deficits in others, which should be cleared using herbs, acupuncture and massage.

In fact, there is an almost *total* lack of agreement on the same disease between different forms of complementary medicine. Only for a very few alternative treatments is there any evidence of efficacy.[135] None of them are completely free of risk.[136] And while physicians can distinguish fact from fiction, patients are not easily able to make sense of conflicting theories.

This does not, however, seem to put people off. Over half of Americans use traditional medicines for various skin-related conditions,[137] whilst Europeans push this rate even higher, and in Africa they are accepted near unanimously.

So, let's briefly review which of the complementary medicines may be effective for vitiligo.

A NECESSARY WORD of Caution

Some of the most powerful drugs – atropine, morphine and quinine, among many – are derived from plants, much like popular herbal supplements. So it's no surprise that natural remedies often interact with prescription drugs in many ways.[138]

When taken concurrently, two medicines with similar therapeutic action can increase drug activity beyond its safe limit. The same is true in reverse, as two medicines can *reduce* each other's effectiveness, or even result in an unexpected toxicity.

For instance, Gingko biloba can improve vitiligo symptoms,

support memory and cardiovascular system, but in high doses it can interfere with around 500 drugs and may affect blood clotting.

Potency of natural remedies depends on biochemical composition, which can vary with age, climate, variety, and soil. It varies even within the same consumer brand because of the season when plants were gathered. (I'm not even talking about the sham products that flood online stores with *who-knows-what* ingredients.) Therefore, the resultant dose and composition of these natural remedies may be truly unpredictable. Adverse interactions with prescription drugs may quickly escalate to life-threatening situations.

TIP: You don't have to choose between conventional and alternative therapy. They can often work well alongside each other. Look for herbal medicines in standardized formulations with instructions for use. Tell your doctor and complementary therapist about all drugs and natural remedies that you are taking regularly.

42

HEALERS AND SHAMANS

C*uraderos* are present-day healers in the Amazon region believed to be at the end of a millennia-long chain of traditional medical knowledge. They possess notions, to a remarkable extent, of therapeutic and restricted use, toxicity, deadliness, and interactions among many plants. I know, as I have met them:

Cezario grabs a glass pebble and puts it over a pulsating artery on my forearm. He lights a candle and half-closes his eyes while staring at the light reflections on the pebble's surface, before chatting about things that are seemingly well above his level of education. In his broken Spanish, he talks of inflammation in the nerves, cells attacking other cells in my skin and blood, toxins in my stomach and many other things I can barely understand.

Cezario is a shaman in Ecuadorian *Oriente*. He is also a healer and chief of several families from the Shuar tribe that live in the basin of Rio Napo, in the middle of nowhere. You can only get there by canoe – navigating endless water passages through rainforest covering a vast area between the Andes, Columbia and Peru.

It was my second visit to Cezario in three years. An expert guide from a Quito-based *Nemo Galapagos Latin Tour* company had traded with Shuar families before, and agreed to drop me off at their place and, hopefully, pick me up a week later. The Shuar were once the region's most ferocious tribespeople, known for centuries as the 'headhunters of the Amazon.' Descendants of these fierce warriors were recently forced away from their native territory by oil drilling and the land contamination that comes with it.

That week I was living with tribespeople in the rainforest, following a strict diet of rice, plantains and herbal drinks. Three times a day I also drank a smelly mixture made from local plants that would – the shaman assured me – cleanse my stomach and balance energy in my organs.

Sometimes at night, Cezario would invite me to join a ritual around the fireplace with fellow tribesmen, where he would share with me *natem* – more widely known as *ayahuasca*[139] – the most potent natural psychedelic brew known to man. He uses *ayahuasca* as a sort of diagnostic tool to discover the roots of illness in his patients, before prescribing remedies for their conditions.

During one of these rituals Cezario delivered his verdict: sadly, he couldn't heal my white spots completely, but told me the disease would stop eating my skin. Indeed, my actively spreading vitiligo came to a complete halt over the next few weeks and remained stable for more than a decade.

Throughout many generations, the Shuar, Huaorani and other local tribes of the upper Amazon's Quichuas people have made profound advances in plant medicine. Much of this indigenous knowledge is not preserved anywhere in writing, and is likely to disappear within a generation. This would be a grave loss.

But the situation is beginning to change. I gave a lecture on ethno-botanical treatments at a VRF Master Class on vitiligo a couple of years ago. It was held hundreds of miles downstream from my early endeavors – in Manaus, the capital of Brazil's Amazon state. We spoke at length with Prof. Sinésio Talhari and his colleagues about a new research project aimed at evaluating indigenous plant medicine and shamanic treatment protocols. Our goal is now to create the bridge between traditional and modern medicine – between shamans and scientists – to find new treatments for vitiligo.

43

TRADITIONAL MEDICINES OF LATIN AMERICA

Since the dawn of human civilization, rainforest plants have been used to treat and alleviate symptoms of what we call autoimmune disorders and inflammatory conditions, including vitiligo, psoriasis, arthritis, lupus, kidney problems and malignant tumors.

Turning to the forest for the next miracle treatment is hardly a new practice. Aspirin first came from willow tree bark and novocaine comes from the coca plant. In fact, a quarter of modern pharmaceuticals are derived from one of 80,000-plus rainforest plants.

Out of those, two plants are particularly well-suited to treating vitiligo:

Polipodium leukotomos

This tropical fern is native to the Honduran rainforests but can be found throughout the South American tropics and the Caribbean. In Brazil, the common name is *samambaia*. In Mexico and other Spanish-speaking countries of the region, the plant is known as *calaguala*.

Several studies have demonstrated a significant effect of the fern on facial vitiligo.[140] Participants were given 250 mg tablets thrice-times daily in combination with NB-UVB, twice-weekly for six months. Most patients reported a substantial repigmentation in the head and neck area, which more pronounced in people with lighter skin – Fitzpatrick types II and III.

There is very little information available about possible side effects of *Polypodium leucotomos*. It may cause an upset stomach in some people. On the positive side, it could reduce reddening – the rate at which skin burns in sunlight – and guard skin from sun damage on a deeper cellular level. It is rapidly absorbed and provides protection that lasts for two to three hours after ingestion, but should not be considered as a replacement for a sunscreen and protective clothing.

Pyrostegia venusta

This neotropical evergreen vine is widespread in Brazil – growing in fields, by the sea, on woodland edges and along roadsides. Popularly known as *cipó-de-são-joão*, meaning flame vine, this species is cultivated due to its outstanding ornamental features, and for use in traditional medicine.

The leaves and stems are used for coughs, bronchitis, flus and colds, while its flowers are used in the treatment of vitiligo. Several pre-clinical studies have confirmed the hyperpigmenting activities of *Pyrostegia venusta,* but side effects, if any, remain unknown.[141]

44

TRADITIONAL MEDICINES OF INDIA

The roots of traditional Indian medicine reach deep into ancient knowledge. The largest branch of this tree is Ayurveda. Others include naturopathy, Siddha medicine, Unani and yoga. A 2,000-year old Ayurvedic text, *Charaka Samhita*, describes vitiligo as *svitra* or *kilasa*.

In Ayurveda, life is the union of body, mind, senses and soul. The primary emphasis is on disease prevention and promoting longevity. It is helpful in chronic, metabolic, and stress-related conditions early in the disease manifestation, before extensive tissue and organ damage has occurred. Frankly, vitiligo is not high on this list.

Treatment for vitiligo begins with calming the imbalanced body energies and restoring digestion. *Psoralea corylifolia*, *Semicarpus anacardium* or *Ficus hispida* are administered as photosensitizers, three hours before graded sun exposure. *Curcuma longa*, *Eclipta alba* or *Acasia catachu* are used to redress blood morbidity. In the case of fast-spreading disease, *Ras Manikya*, *Taal Sindur* or *Sameer Pannag Ras* are used as immunosuppressants to stop its progression. Stubborn patches are camouflaged with the paste made from mehndi leaves, or a lotion made from the root of *Plumbago Zylanica*.

Side effects of these herbal preparations are rarely reported in full, if at all. Pharmacological evidence suggests there could be toxicity issues – similar to those discussed in the PUVA chapter – and in rare cases the possibility of renal failure or cancer.

Ayurvedic medicine also acknowledges the risks involved in using arsenic and mercury – common ingredients in these preparations. One out of five Ayurvedic herbal medicine products found in Asian food stores in the USA reportedly contains harmful levels of heavy metals.[142] Worse, some of them are specifically recommended for pediatric use. In England, a third of all Ayurvedic medicines sampled have dangerous amounts of heavy metal content, while in India the same is seen in two-thirds of products.

45

TRADITIONAL MEDICINES OF CHINA

Several millennia of growth have transformed Chinese medicine into a remarkable field of therapy. The body's health is defined as a balance of two opposing yet complimentary forces – Yin and Yang – in every organ, and an uninterrupted flow of the vital force Qi throughout the body. Imbalance of these forces manifests itself as an illness. Symptoms may appear on the skin, mediated by the blood, but cause is always rooted in internal organs.

Throughout Asia, practitioners of traditional Chinese medicine combine herbal medicines with various mind and body practices, such as acupuncture, *qi gong* and *tai chi*. In the United States, people think of it largely as herbal therapy.

Three different ancient Chinese medical terms match the description of vitiligo – *Bai-Dian*, *Bai-Bo-Feng* and *Ban-Bo* – with the two most common syndromes being:

- liver and kidney deficiency, and
- Qi stagnation and blood stasis.

In accordance with this classification, generations of traditional Chinese medicine practitioners have been prescribing herbs first to revitalize liver and kidney, then to reduce blood inflammation and to expel 'wind evil.'

Gao et al recently conducted a thorough analysis of the Chinese literature and international databases to determine effective remedies for vitiligo.[143] Among 163 known formula prescriptions – each containing between three and 25 herbs – the three most popular were *Tong-Qiao-Huo-Xue* decoction, *Xiao-Yao* powder and *Si-Wu* decoction. Three of the twelve most common herbs include *Angelica sinensis*, *Ligusticum wallichii* and *Tribulus terrestris*.

Like conventional medicines, traditional Chinese herbal medicines may also cause side effects, trigger allergic reactions, or interfere with prescription drugs. Many manufacturers do not always follow tradition: at least a third of products commercially available in California contain undeclared pharmaceuticals or heavy metals in unsafe concentrations and are often mislabeled.[144,145]

Ginkgo Biloba

GINKGO BILOBA EXTRACT seems to be a simple, relatively safe and fairly effective therapy for arresting the progression of vitiligo.

Ginkgo is a large tree with fan-shaped leaves, normally reaching a height of 66–115 ft (20–35 m) in temperate regions, and can live up to one thousand years. It is native to parts of China, Japan, and Korea. The ginkgo family is a living fossil – it has been around since before the dinosaurs – but *Ginkgo biloba* is the only surviving species of the original *Ginkgo*.

Today's ginkgo trees are descendants of the ones planted in the gardens of ancient Buddhist temples in China and Japan. They have been grown in Europe since around 1730 and in the United States since around 1784. Ginkgoes are almost extinct in the wild nowadays but flourish along the Fifth Avenue and other streets of New York city. They have an extraordinary ability to survive the heat, the snows, the hurricanes, the pollution, and other extremes of the mega-city.

Ginkgo extracts have been employed medicinally for a variety of ways. They have been used to improve blood flow to the brain, thereby enhancing cognitive performance and protecting against Alzheimer's disease. It is considered helpful immediately following strokes, in treatment of eye and ear disorders, skin health management, blood pressure control, multiple sclerosis and dozens of other conditions.

In similar trials conducted by Parsad[146] in India and Szczurko [147] in Canada, participants were given 40 mg or 60 mg of the standardized extract. People were instructed to take one oral capsule three and two times per day, respectively, 10 minutes before a meal. Disease activity stopped in nearly all patients with facial vitiligo over the course of 12 weeks, and marked repigmentation was evident in half of them after six months.

The ease of taking an oral pill, the relatively low cost, and the low frequency of adverse reactions, make Ginkgo biloba use tempting for vitiligo management. There is no consensus among specialists on the maximum daily dosage, with suggestions ranging from 80 to 600 mg/day. Manufacturers recommend a twice-daily intake of 120 mg of a standardized leaf extract with a meal, and a daily dose of 240 mg appears to be safe.[148]

Ginkgo biloba may have side effects, which include stomach complaints, dyspepsia, and nausea. However, it has potential interactions with many prescription drugs, including blood thinners, high blood pressure medications, and antidepressants. Check with your doctor before starting with Gingko biloba therapy – especially if you are regularly taking aspirin, warfarin, ibuprofen, ticlopidine, azpazolam, digoxin, diltiazem, haloperidol, trazodone, nicardipine, nifedipine, omerprazole, thiazide diuretics, tolbutamide, or valproate.

TIP: Do not use traditional medicines as a replacement for conventional treatment, or as a reason to postpone seeing a dermatologist. With very few exceptions, conventional treatment stops vitiligo progression faster, and provides longer and more stable repigmentation with manageable side effects.

46

VITAMINS AND DIET

I n simple terms, autoimmune diseases like vitiligo result in communication breakdown at a cellular level, when an out-of-control immune system begins to attack healthy, but stressed out cells. White lesions on the skin are just the tip of the iceberg. Much of what's going on below the surface is still a mystery.

Nonetheless, and often with the best intentions, many 'experts' produce all kinds of dietary recommendations for vitiligo. Their pseudo-scientific jargon is pervasive, making it difficult to separate fact from fiction.

It does not mean there is no possible link between vitiligo and nutrition, but the vitamin-vs-diet-vs-disease debate is too complex for simple generalizations. It changes and depends on the nutrients under scrutiny and the individual's health condition. And one shouldn't expect a 50 mg vitamin pill to have the same effect in a 100-pound woman as a 200-pound man.

A Double-Edged Sword

Many supermarkets and drug stores devote an entire aisle to

nutritional supplements, so it's no wonder people turn to vitamins to help their vitiligo. Better cover all bases, as the thinking
goes. Alas, there is still no firm evidence that taking a vitamin will
work for vitiligo in general, or for its specific subtype. While it
may support your health in some ways, it could hurt it in others.

It's actually very difficult to make educated statements about
vitamins, as their mechanism of action is not fully understood.
Natural antioxidants like vitamin C, vitamin E, carotenoids, and
polyphenols like flavonoids, are generally seen to be beneficial
components. Their anti-oxidative properties are often claimed to
be responsible for various beneficial health effects. However, at
higher doses or under certain conditions these anti-oxidants may
exert toxic, pro-oxidant activities.[149]

Vitamin C may therefore both promote and hinder vitiligo
lesion growth, depending on the dose and existing level of oxidative stress in a patient's skin. High doses of vitamin C – if not
properly quenched by vitamin E – could result in an increased
oxidant burden.[150]

Take, as another example, vitamin B_{12}. This vitamin is often
deficient in vitiligo patients compared to the general population.
(It is also deficient in about 80% of vegans.) But supplementation
of vitamin B_{12} is necessary *only* in those vitiligo patients who also
have pernicious anemia. Even then it should be injected rather
than taken orally, because it cannot be efficiently absorbed
through the stomach.[151] Dieticians and physicians thus recommend megadoses of oral vitamin B_{12} medication – but only as a
cost-saving and more comfortable alternative to intramuscular injections – without much regard to actual effect it has on the
body. Medications such as metformin (Glucophage) or antacids
can further impair B_{12} absorption.

Vitamin D is another example of uncertainty. A large part of
the population is seemingly deficient in this vitamin, but this
rather questions the 'norm' itself. Even the nudists in Florida
have low vitamin D! Low levels of vitamin D can also be a marker

of susceptibility to other autoimmune disease. Vitiligo patients may be deficient in this vitamin for many reasons, but this doesn't mean that vitamin D supplementation is likely to help their condition.

Organic vs Western Diet

Time and again, we hear that healthy eating beats taking supplements. It has been repeated so often that 'natural' and 'organic' have positive connotations in our minds, whereas 'manufactured' or 'synthetic' have negative ones.

But this rule is bunk – much like the opposite claim that your body needs multi-vitamins to supplement a standard 'Western' diet, as soil depletion and industrialized farming have deprived natural foods of essential microelements. Proponents add that our food is a mess of pesticides, heavy metals, poisons, GMO and a bunch of unknown compounds.

The truth, of course, isn't so clear cut. Many foods found in Western supermarkets – milk, eggs, cereals and salt, to name a few – are already fortified with micronutrients you may lack. They *already* act as food supplements. By the same token, many vitamins have natural and synthetic forms, and make necessary microelements accessible to people with restricted food intake, for religious, medicinal or a mixture of other reasons.

It is probably a good idea to support our gut microbiota by incorporating fermented foods such as kefir, yogurt or sauerkraut. These are rich in nutrients, enzymes and healthy bacteria to help balance the immune system.

Gluten-free Diet

Gluten is a storage protein in wheat, rye, and barley that puffs up when baked with yeast. It may promote inflammation and intestinal damage in the 0.7% of the population with celiac disease. Children and infants are most likely to show signs of a wheat allergy or gluten intolerance, which are different conditions with similar symptoms.

In all my years at VRF, I witnessed only a handful of cases when vitiligo improved after gluten restriction. If you are wondering about gluten in your child's diet, or someone in your family has a history of food allergies, it is best to get a confirmed diagnosis before you start messing with diet. Two to three months of a gluten-restricted diet is enough to see if it can help your vitiligo.

BOTTOM LINE: In theory, supplements or diets could work for vitiligo — if we actually knew what is necessary. Some commercially available multivitamins may also help a little, but probably not a lot.

47

CLIMATOTHERAPY

The Dead Sea is the saltiest body of water in the world, and also the lowest point on the Earth's surface, dipping to 430 meters below sea level amidst a parched desert shared by Jordan, Israel and the West Bank. It's called 'dead' as no fish or aquatic organisms can live in the water, which are seven-times the average ocean salinity.

It is said that Cleopatra believed in the mystical healing powers of the 'Bahr Lut,' as it was also known, and built the world's first spa resort here. Two thousand years later, scientists have confirmed the effectiveness of Dead Sea therapy for vitiligo, psoriasis and other conditions.[152]

Therapy consists of graded sun exposure combined with Dead Sea baths. Therapeutic factors are mostly attributed to the unique spectrum of sunlight at the bottom of the basin. The extremely low altitude – it is the lowest place on Earth – creates an extremely high atmospheric pressure with a high concentration of oxygen. Thick air, rich with bromine and other minerals, blocks the harmful type A (UVA) ultraviolet rays, while allowing therapeutic type B (UVB) rays to reach your skin.

The dose of UVB is more important than the length of sun

exposure. As the sunlight properties change within the day and throughout the year, my recommendations below should be individually adjusted by a knowledgeable vitiligo specialist.

A typical daily treatment routine begins between 7 and 8 a.m. with a 15-minute swim. Minerals that make these waters deadly to fish, make it a prescription treatment for vitiligo. It's fun to float effortlessly in the water – in fact, it's impossible to sink! Just don't put your head in, as the salt can burn your eyes.

Prof. Karin Schallreuter recommends the use of pseudocatalase cream over the whole body and sunbathing naked at the gender-conscious solarium. The proprietary synthetic formulation is believed to speed up the initiation of repigmentation, though it is entirely optional.[153,154] The follow-up, low-dose UVB protocol, and supportive community helps patients improve quality of life once they get back home.

The swim and sunbathing procedure is repeated at around 4 p.m. As the treatment progresses, the daily sun exposure is gradually increased from minutes to an hour. A therapeutic goal is to achieve a sustained pink color on white patches, without them turning red. Patients are advised to protect themselves with clothing or sunscreens from extra sun exposure that is not included in their treatment protocol.

Three weeks is the minimum overall period for climatotherapy. The longer the stay at the Dead Sea, the better the result. Repigmentation begins after one or two weeks, then major improvement is often seen towards the end of the fourth week. Repigmentation usually continues after returning home for another six to eight weeks. While facial vitiligo responds and regains color quickly, repigmentation of hands and feet will require several trips to the Dead Sea.

The best treatment period is from March to late October. However, June, July and August are too hot for many to explore the natural wonders and rich history of the region in between the procedures. Whilst I was there, I enjoyed gym and sports during the day, stayed the night in the Wadi Rum desert, visited the ancient fortress of Masada, and had a trip to the unforgettable Petra.

Dr. Marco Harari, a recognized expert on the Dead Sea climatotherapy, concludes: "More than four decades after being studied, it can be considered now as a natural and simple dermatological treatment, highly effective and free of side effects."[155]

Therapy at the Dead Sea is the only treatment that's safe for nearly *all* vitiligo patients – regardless of age, and including pregnant and nursing women. Rare contraindications include photosensitive skin disorders, renal insufficiency, acute infection, and severe movement disability. One should be aware that ultraviolet light is carcinogenic, an important cause of skin cancer.

Home Resort

The combination of balneotherapy and artificial phototherapy has been proven effective thousands of miles away from the Dead Sea, in Kazakhstan. According to Dr. Kassymkhanova, a warm bath with Dead Sea salts 1 ounce (30 g) per 10 gallons (40 l) for 15 minutes prior to every UVB phototherapy session significantly improves treatment outcomes.[156]

Fifteen balneotherapy procedures in combination with the ongoing UVB treatment seems to kick-start repigmentation, even in difficult to treat lesions. This kind of re-created climatotherapy is ideally combined with home-based UVB treatment. No Dead Sea travel needed, but you'll miss all the fun that comes with it.

MYTH BUSTED: 'Vitiligo is incurable, so you just have to live with it.' Only half true. Treatments have the potential to provide years of vitiligo-free life.

PART X

CAMOUFLAGE

~

"I'd far rather be happy than right any day." Douglas
Adams,
   The Hitchhiker's Guide to the Galaxy

48

MAKEUP FROM MALE PERSPECTIVE

My own relationship with makeup begun with my first job at a big investment firm. I tried to mask my vitiligo spots with a rudimentary mix of cosmetics I found abandoned by my ex-girlfriend in the bathroom. It was an unflattering experience. In the early 1990s, few men – unless they were off to a Halloween party – would think of wearing makeup without feeling painfully awkward.

Fortunately, I soon moved up to the PR department with a lax dress code and turtle-necks became a year-round staple of my wardrobe. For the next twenty-odd years I have sporadically, and rather unsuccessfully, tried dozens of cosmetic products. I finally stopped hiding my vitiligo spots after the launch of Vitiligo Research Foundation.

I won't pretend therefore I know much about cosmetic camouflage. And no matter how many advances I make in makeup use, I will lag forever behind a school-age girl who just started playing with it.

So, I think my only use here is to provide a quick look at vitiligo camouflage options from a man's perspective. Rather than being a lousy guide to the galaxy of cosmetic products, this part is intended to simply mark a starting point for beginners like myself.

49

COSMETIC CAMOUFLAGE

There are two basic approaches to cosmetic camouflage for vitiligo. Concealing is used to cover wide body areas using creamy products of a variety of shades. Color correcting is used to disguise skin lesions only, using products that yield a tan-like skin appearance.

Traditional Preparations: Fast and Cheap

Liquid dyes like henna and traditional Indian preparations are fast and cheap camouflage options, but these are their sole benefits. Getting a good color match is very difficult and the pigment is easily washed or rubbed off.

Dihydroxyacetone: Slow, Safe and Lasting

Men have been conditioned for generations to believe that makeup is for girls. That's why fake tan – rather than makeup – probably comes first to most men's minds when needing to cover a nasty vitiligo spot.

Most of these 'sunless tanning' products contain an active

ingredient called dihydroxyacetone, abbreviated as DHA. When applied to the skin, DHA causes a safe, slow chemical reaction in the surface cells that creates a transient darkening effect. There should be no surprise that DHA creams of 3%-6% concentrations are popular across the world as an effective way to camouflage vitiligo lesions.[157]

DHA is easy to apply and is neither dirty nor greasy, but the result is highly dependent on skin preparation and application technique. Possible residues from soaps or detergents must first be wiped off the skin with hydroalcoholic toner, allowing the DHA to interact with amino acids in the skin. Also, moisturizing the skin before and after DHA application with a damp cotton pad will make the recolored area look smoother.

The simulated pigmentation normally begins to appear within an hour of application, and the darkening effect may peak after about four to eight hours. The intensity of the color depends on the thickness and roughness of the skin, and several applications every few hours may be required to achieve a deep, dark color. Thicker layers and more frequent reapplications are required to maintain color on the face, than on the hands or feet. Perfect color matching and seamless blending with the surrounding skin is therefore difficult to obtain. Depending on the body area and amount of repeat applications, the color effect will last until the dead skin cells rub off – usually after five or six days.

Dihydroacetone is generally approved by the FDA for use in self-tanning products, except for on the area around the eyes and on the lips. Unlike most cosmetic products, DHA does not block UV radiation, so fake tanned skin still needs full sun protection. Similarly, DHA will *not* interfere with UVB phototherapy and thus doesn't have to be removed before the procedure and re-applied later – a huge timesaver for those using camouflage during light therapy.

AN EXCELLENT CONCEALER for vitiligo is produced by Zanderm – a family-owned company based in Brooklyn, NY, USA.[158] Its flagship product was born from an idea that James Adelson and Sara Frankel had while working together on a tan line corrector for a cosmetic company. As Jim and Sara continued to perfect DHA-based darkening solution for different skin colors, they realized this could also work for vitiligo patients.

The team went through all the trials and tribulations of new cosmetic product development, and I was an early tester of every new batch. The real challenge was how to create an immediate 'wow!' effect with a subtle process that requires several hours for full strength – achievable on all kinds of skin types and body parts – while delivering a decent shelf life in various climate zones.

DHA-based concealers are water and smudge-proof, which makes them perfect for use on hands and feet. They don't limit your clothing choices, as the color is formed in the upper skin layer, so does not come off like regular makeup. They also allow skin to breathe, therefore concealer does not need to be washed off every day.

Perfecting application techniques may take a week or two, but the convenience and discretion of a concealer pen is worth this small effort.

Medical Makeup: Perfect but Costly

At every cosmetics store the choice seems endless. There are a myriad of brands with various products and formulations available for medical makeup.[159] Sadly, gender-conscious and overly nice salespeople are seldom trained in the intricacies of makeup application for medical conditions, so can offer little assistance. One of the other reasons I have never considered makeup for my vitiligo an appealing option is because it stains clothing, especially shirt neck collars.

However, the proliferation of male makeup and concealers since the turn of the century – now called 'grooming products' – has again made me curious about cosmetic alternatives to vitiligo treatment.

The best concealers on the market today can mask facial vitiligo and blend in effortlessly with natural skin tone. As an added benefit, they can also remove nearly every sign of a well-lived life from your skin. Cosmetic camouflage – put on with a simple twist-up stick or a heavy-duty set – lasts a whole day with a single application.

Using a Band-Aid theory for camouflaging skin discoloration, professional makeup artists achieve amazing results.[160] But when done badly (by guys like me), the results can be downright disastrous. Camouflage may also require maintenance during the day, unlike DHA-based concealers.

The biggest stumbling block to men's use of cosmetic camouflage, however, may be the sheer time and effort it takes to learn the process and then apply makeup properly.

50

TATTOOS

You may remember that Lee Thomas – our TV presenter friend – had his first sign of vitiligo, a white spot on his hand, tattooed black to match his skin. Yet his relief was short-lived, as the disease quickly depigmented the surrounding areas – creating an island of artificial pigment that served as a desolate reminder of his life before vitiligo.

With permanent cosmetics, ink is injected into the upper layers of the skin using a traditional tattoo coil, pen or rotary machines, or hand devices. Actually, tattoos aren't permanent: they fade and change color, which requires a periodic color refreshing. Tattoo longevity varies from person to person, depending on the type of ink pigment, sun exposure and their lifestyle.

More than fifty different pigments and shades are currently in use for permanent tattoos and makeup. Yet *none of them* are approved by the U.S. Food and Drug Administration for injection into skin.

Whatever the motive, possible tattoo complications include infection, scars or granulomas, keloid formation, allergic reactions and even interference with MRI procedures. When tattoo ink is applied to the skin, most of it remains firmly lodged there, but some pigments ride the bloodstream to lymph nodes, the liver and further afield.

There are also risks linked to tattoo removal. It is a painstaking process and the consequences of how pigments break down after laser treatment is not yet understood. However, it's clear that some tattoo removal procedures leave permanent scarring.

TIP: The unpredictable nature of the disease and adverse reactions following tattoo removal are the key arguments against permanent camouflage.

PART XI

DEPIGMENTATION

~

51

FIGHT FIRE WITH FIRE

In March 2010, detectives from Los Angeles Police Department investigating Michael Jackson's death found 19 tubes of hydroquinone 8% lotion, 18 tubes of Benoquin® 20% cream, and a tube with BQ/KA/RA (Benoquin® 8%, Kojic acid 1%, and retinoic acid 0.025%) mixture in his house. These are all common ingredients in skin lightening products and it didn't take long for social and mainstream media to switch into overdrive.

For years the late King Of Pop has been widely criticized for his use of bleaching medications and chemical peels, which were seen to be part of an overly extravagant lifestyle. As Michael Jackson's skin color became ever paler, it bewildered and angered many of his fans.

Yet while he appeared to be turning to white, his skin was actually becoming translucent – devoid of *any* color. During an Oprah show in 1993 Jackson said his skin started to change sometime after *Thriller*, released a decade earlier. Vitiligo evidently progressed beyond his ability to cover it with make-up. Reluctantly, he switched strategy and resorted to the ultimate weapon in the vitiligo arsenal – depigmentation. In a later interview with

Larry King on CNN, Dr. Arnold Klein, Jackson's dermatologist acknowledged that: "We basically used creams that would even out the same color and we destroyed the remaining pigment cells."

WHEN A FEW ISLANDS of natural skin color vividly stand out against a sea of milky white vitiligo, depigmentation is often the only option to create a flawless look.[161] Depigmentation gradually removes the remaining pigment forever, by destroying or deactivating melanocytes. This medical procedure essentially causes irreversible vitiligo, and should *only* be used when all other options have failed.

The first line in depigmentation therapy is commonly assigned to chemical agents. For fast and easily available color removal, cryotherapy should be considered first. Delicate and precision work at a higher cost is reserved for lasers.

Patients with active vitiligo have better chances for depigmentation than with stable disease. Young onset age and the presence of Koebner phenomenon are good prognostic factors for therapy.

The decision to go colorless should not be taken lightly. Complete depigmentation may take several months, depending on the therapy of choice, and will result in extreme skin sensitivity to sunlight and ultraviolet radiation. Life-long sun protection will be necessary to prevent repigmentation upon treatment cessation. Social ramifications and cultural stigmas may also arise.

52

DEPIGMENTATION AGENTS

A variety of topical depigmenting agents are used clinically, with varying degrees of success. One of the most effective pharmacological formulations is a combination of hydroquinone with other agents; however, its use is associated with frequent adverse reactions. Cosmetic depigmenting agents discussed in Chapter *Snow White Syndrome* are generally safer but less effective than their pharmacological counterparts.

Ether of Hydroquinone: MBEH and MMEH

Monobenzyl ether of hydroquinone (MBEH) is the only depigmentation treatment for extensive vitiligo that has been approved by the FDA in the U.S. It is commercially available under the trade name Benoquin®, and as custom compounds at local pharmacies.

Different concentrations of MBEH can be used on different body parts – for example 5% on the neck, 10% on the face, and 20% on the arms and legs. MBEH in 30% and 40% formulations may also be used to treat difficult areas that resist weaker concentrations, like elbows and knees, over the course of three to four months. Keep in mind that custom compounds should be kept in a refrigerator and typically used within six months.

A thin layer of MBEH cream should be applied twice or thrice-daily to the target areas, except for eyelids and skin surrounding body cavities. Hair, eyebrow and eyelash areas may be resistant to depigmentation and therefore may require a combination approach.[162] Partial depigmentation is usually achieved after one to four months of cream use. However, it may take up to 12 months for complete removal of color from the skin.

Sun protection with SPF30+ is necessary from the beginning of depigmentation therapy to avoid spontaneous repigmentation on the exposed skin – something that is not uncommon.[163] Safety data on the affect of MBEH on pregnant or breastfeeding women, and children under 12 years, is unclear due to the restrictive nature of clinical trials.

Side effects are mostly mild, but MBEH may cause depigmentation *away* from the application site – even on another part of the body. This might be a problem for patients with lighter skin types who are seeking depigmentation only of cosmetically sensitive areas, like the face and neckline. There have also been reports of depigmentation effecting others through close proximity to the cream user, so patients must avoid contact of MBEH-covered skin with the skin of others.

Patients on MBEH therapy sometimes complain about skin irritation and contact dermatitis. If blistering, scaling, dry skin or swelling of treated sites occurs, treatment should be paused and a topical steroid applied to the area, then restarted with a lower concentration when the problem subsides. In rare cases, a blue-black skin discoloration can occur after MBEH use.[164]

You should also be aware of Monomethyl ether of hydroquinone (MMEH), also known as 4-methoxyphenol or mequinol. This has similar properties to MBEH, but is weaker and has milder side effects. A disadvantage of MMEH is the longer treatment period compared to MBEH cream.

Phenol Solution: Experience Required

Phenol solution is a cheap, widely available, fast-acting yet debatable option for depigmentation.[165,166] It should be used cautiously, just on small areas and only by experienced physicians.

Phenol does not cause destruction of melanocytes. Instead, it compromises their ability to produce pigment. Hence, spontaneous repigmentation is a greater concern with this treatment.

Side effects are less than with MBEH. In high concentrations phenol can cause severe chemical burns and heart arrhythmias. Cardiac risk is too concerning, especially since phenol could be used on large body areas. Other risks of phenol use may include scarring, irregular areas of pigmentation and depigmentation, and herpes simplex virus infection that occurs with localized blistering.

Laser: Costly but Effective

As we discussed in Part Eight, lasers with 308-311 nm wavelength are regularly used to stimulate melanocytes and induce repigmentation in vitiligo. A different category of lasers – with a faster pulse frequency and a higher wavelength – is used to reduce pigmentation, or to remove color from the skin completely.

Q-switched lasers, such as the ruby (694 nm), alexandrite (755 nm) and Nd:YAG (532 nm and 1064 nm) work by selectively destroying melanin and melanocytes.[167] Lasers may be used alone or in combination with MBEH or MMEH for better results. Q-switched laser therapy is effective in approximately half of patients, and may require up to 10 sessions for complete depigmentation.[168]

Main advantages of lasers over pharmacological agents include speed, efficiency and safety. Lasers can be used on sensitive areas where chemical agents cannot be applied. They don't create the side effects associated with topical therapies, like redness, burning, itching or scarring.

The main disadvantages of using lasers for depigmentation are high cost, select availability and the possible recurrence of pigmentation. Laser treatment may also be painful, so local anesthesia is often required.

Cryotherapy: Fast and Cost-effective

Therapy with liquid nitrogen is another cost-effective tactic to clear color from small areas that are resistant to MBEH. Nitrogen at -196°C is briefly applied to the skin lesion with a spray, or a cotton-tipped applicator. This simple procedure may be repeated two to three times at four to six week intervals, until complete depigmentation occurs.

The main advantages of cryotherapy are the wide availability of liquid nitrogen at dermatology clinics, and a predictable depigmentation process. Compared to the laser therapy, cryotherapy requires longer downtime between sessions, but takes fewer sessions and is faster overall.

On the flip side, cryotherapy is not suited for treatment of large areas in one sitting, as irregular patterns of pigmentation and depigmentation may randomly occur. The cryotherapy procedure may cause pain and the discomfort will remain for some time afterwards. Undesirable effects may include scarring, persistent or recurrent skin lesions, thus necessitating further treatments.

PART XII

WRAPPING UP

~

53

CATCH-22: BREAK THE VICIOUS CYCLE

I have a fuzzy memory of a day in summer camp when I was a goalie in a soccer game. A six-year-old, I was no match for older kids on the field and was left to defend our team's bottom line. Weathered goal posts seemed like half-a-mile away, totally out of reach. Imagine my horror when, with the opposition bearing down on me, I smashed into a post and a piece of rusty metal pierced my leg like a fish hook. Several months later a small white lesion appeared around the injury site. It wasn't just a Koebner phenomenon – as some might argue after reading previous chapters – because I had previously bruised my skin many times while learning to ride a bike and all of them healed without a trace.

This stressful image of my skin hanging on a piece of rusty metal has been embedded in my mind, like a fly in amber, ever since. It may have caused a chain reaction, which ultimately wrecked the intricate web of forces that keep my body safe.

WE HAVE all heard that stress is toxic to our immune system. Stressful events in childhood can derange the basic function of our immune cells and take a costly long-term toll on our health. Overwhelmed by unrelenting psychological stressors at work, irregular sleep patterns, unhealthy diets, and daily exposure to hazardous chemicals, our immune system goes into constant overdrive mode and never gets a chance to recover. Immune cells become so beleaguered that they start to attack healthy tissues, causing a variety of autoimmune conditions – including vitiligo.

A meta-analysis by Prof. Schwartz shows evidence that patients with vitiligo are also prone to low self-esteem and depressive symptoms.[169] The degree of depigmentation directly correlates with psychological impact and even suicidal thoughts.[170]

This brings us to a Catch-22 situation: emotional stress can cause vitiligo, which can lead to more stress that sparks vitiligo. How can we break this vicious circle? By keeping a low baseline of emotional stress, we can protect our immune system from episodes of erratic behavior. Regular meditation, prayer, cognitive therapy, or simply strolling through the woods can unplug us from the strains of modern life, and lower stress hormone levels.

54

AVOID KNOWN CHEMICAL TRIGGERS

I t is important to remember there are multiple factors involved in vitiligo onset. On the one hand, our skin is remarkably porous and our internal organs are adept at absorbing toxic materials from our environment. On the other, our living spaces are stacked with hazardous substances – both known and unmarked.

People genetically predisposed to vitiligo can reach that noxious threshold at which the disease becomes active with just one wrong choice. Yet, you don't even have to possess a genetic predisposition for vitiligo to unleash killer immune cells that hunt melanocytes down.

Trying to avoid known chemical triggers and immune system disruptors can be overwhelming and frustrating. It seems like anything you touch, inhale or eat carries health risks. Cosmetic products contain a disturbing number of harsh chemicals. Some hair dyes and whitening creams are known to cause vitiligo. Wet rubber shoes leak contact irritants that may cause leukoderma. Even homeopathic treatments are loaded with heavy metals and toxins.

Protect your skin and immune system with everyday choices.

Buy greener house cleaning products and cosmetics. Drive a few extra miles to shop at an organic food store, or swim at a well-maintained pool. Ask your hairstylist about natural hair dyes. Request material safety data sheets at work. And use your common sense when making any purchase, because each small choice matters.

55

START TREATMENT PROMPTLY

I t often takes years for vitiligo to be properly diagnosed and a lifetime to keep it at bay. There is, sadly, no silver bullet for vitiligo.

Early treatment – ideally, within first three months of lesion detection – increases chances for successful outcomes, but even decades-old lesions can be repigmented with enough patience. White lesions frequently reappear when treatment is discontinued, with relapse occurring in nearly half of all patients within four years of stopping treatment. This relapse can be significantly decreased with supportive phototherapy and other treatments.

Light therapy remains a gold standard, though it is hard to predict precisely who will respond to which type of treatment. About a third of patients are non-respondents (or late respondents, to be exact) and the therapy may take one or two years to restore natural skin color. Dietary supplements and vitamins can mildly enhance phototherapy effectiveness but are incapable of creating a lasting effect on their own.

Meanwhile, researchers are on the hunt for clues to better understand vitiligo and immune systems, with clinical trials for new treatments already on the horizon. As Big Pharma sees signs of substantial progress in this area, there is a race starting to see who will be the first to make a vitiligo drug approved by the U.S. FDA. At the time of writing, thirteen pharmaceutical companies are either funding their own vitiligo research programs, or supporting programs at academic labs.

You can find a study to participate in through ClinicalTrials.gov – the largest database of privately and publicly funded clinical studies from around the world.

56

SUPPLEMENT YOUR WHOLE BODY

Having a specialist who can diagnose disease quickly and accurately, and treat it with the best available medicines is a good thing. But on the downside, Western physicians are neither trained nor paid to go 'upstream' – that is, to the source of the problem. These specialists are also less likely to think of the body as a holistic system – something more common to Eastern medicine and traditional healers. Dermatologists who focus solely on a patient's skin treatment often miss the interconnection between vitiligo and their immune system condition, accompanying diseases, genetic background, environmental factors, and lifestyle.

An essential matter for anyone suffering from vitiligo, or at risk from any autoimmune condition, is to ensure well-balanced nutrition. Our gut is intricately linked to what's happening elsewhere in the body, though much of it remains poorly understood. As if this connection wasn't complex enough, the natural quality of what goes into the stomach – from foods to supplements – is also a subject of great controversy.

I would suggest to begin with home-cooked meals from local

produce and 'anti-autoimmune disease' diet, and to share your progress with your family doctor.

57

NEXT STEPS

Let's liken your next steps in this journey to driving a car. There are many destinations you can drive to – some of them are within reach, some are far away. You may be in a fancy, powerful car – nonetheless if you feel like you have no control over it, then you will be scared and miserable. Yet if you are behind the wheel of your beaten but dependable truck, which you know inside out, then you will feel happy and confident.

So, the trick is to take control over your ride by assuming full responsibility for what happens during your journey. You may not be in control of what's happening on the road, but you are always responsible for how you respond to it. That means accessing proper and regular medical advice is your responsibility. Proper diet for your immune system is your responsibility, too.

There is no shortcut on this journey, but you can set checkpoints along the way and re-evaluate your situation as you move forward. Set small and achievable goals, like first checking your environment for known vitiligo triggers. You must review everything you come into contact with from this perspective. Once you achieve this goal, your confidence level will rise a little bit.

Next, raise the stakes to a higher level. When you go shopping, check every label before handing your hard-earned money to the cashier. Do this long enough and you will start feeling like you have taken control over what goes into your house and your body.

Your next checkpoint is planning your personalized diet, which will send signal to your immune system. Before long, you will have the willpower to get to the following checkpoint and so on. And whether you actually reach your destination or not, you'll be a lot happier, with increased self-esteem and belief in yourself.

AFTERWORD

Whichever track you took through this book, you now have a better overview of vitiligo than 99% of people who live with it, or are helping a family member who has vitiligo. I hope this book answers your questions or touches on your thoughts. If not, let me know and I will either try again or concede the point. And if you'd like to get regular updates, please visit www.vitiligo.tips and subscribe to the newsletter.

Sincerely,

Yan Valle

ABOUT THE AUTHOR

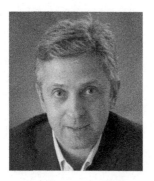

Yan Valle is an author, vitiligo spokesperson and strategist.

As a patient since around six years of age, Yan has gone through every common pitfall known to a person diagnosed with vitiligo: misdiagnosis, years of non-treatment followed by bursts of mistreatment, self-prescription and self-medication, to name a few.

As a professional, Yan went from nearly three decades in the high-tech and business development sector to become Chief Executive Officer of the 501(c)3 non-profit Vitiligo Research Foundation, based in New York, USA.

A frequent lecturer, Yan also serves as a contract professor at the University of Guglielmo Marconi in Rome, Italy. Yan also consults on bio-informatics and the use of real-world data for the next generation of healthcare applications.

Contact Yan via form on the website or by email:

www.vitiligo.tips
info@vitiligo.tips

LINKS AND REFERENCES

1. Lee Thomas, an Emmy Award-winning broadcaster and motivational speaker. Thomas wrote a memoir of his own journey with the skin condition, Turning White. He is also involved with helping other vitiligo sufferers through the Clarity Lee Thomas Foundation. http://www.leethomas.com
2. This story originally aired on Fox 2 Detroit on World Vitiligo Day. https://www.youtube.com/watch?v=AJNQVI7OqFg
3. XX Master Class On Vitiligo and II Winter Consensus Conference http://vrfoundation.org/doctors-page--4/master-classes/roundtable-on-vitiligo-in-rome-december-2016
4. UN International Calendar of Disability Events https://www.un.org/development/desa/disabilities/calendar.html
5. Winnie Harlow official website: http://www.officialwinnieharlow.com
6. World Vitiligo Day, observed on June 25, is global initiative aimed to build global awareness about

vitiligo. This is a day of celebration of our lives and our community. The first World Vitiligo Day was held in 2011 and has since become an annual, global event. Over the years, its purpose has broadened from raising awareness of vitiligo to include recognition of the bullying, social neglect, psychological trauma and disability of millions of people affected by vitiligo. Official website: http://25june.org

7. Winnie Harlow official Instagram https://www.instagram.com/winnieharlow/

8. Ciudad Mitad Del Mundo – Middle of the World City - is a tract of land located 26 km north of the center of capital city Quito in the province of Pichincha, Ecuador. The grounds contain the Monument to the Equator, which highlights the exact location of the equator (from which the country takes its name); they also contain the Museo Etnográfico Mitad del Mundo, a museum about the indigenous ethnography of Ecuador. Wikipedia: https://en.wikipedia.org/wiki/Ciudad_Mitad_del_Mun do

9. Krüger C, Schallreuter KU. A review of the worldwide prevalence of vitiligo in children/adolescents and adults. Int J Dermatol. 2012. 51(10):1206-12 PubMed: https://www.ncbi.nlm.nih.gov/pubmed/22458952

10. Silverberg NB. The Epidemiology of Vitiligo. Curr Derm Rep (2015) 4: 36. https://doi.org/10.1007/s13671-014-0098-6

11. Zhang Y, Cai Y, Shi M, et al. 2016. The Prevalence of Vitiligo: A Meta-Analysis. PLoS ONE11(9): e0163806. https://www.ncbi.nlm.nih.gov/pmc/articles/PMC50389 43/

12. Alkhateeb A, Fain P, Spritz R, et al. Epidemiology of Vitiligo and Associated Autoimmune Diseases in

Caucasian Probands and Their Families. Pigment cell research / sponsored by the European Society for Pigment Cell Research and the International Pigment Cell Society. 2003. 16. 208-14. 10.1034/j.1600-0749.2003.00032.x. http://onlinelibrary.wiley.com/doi/10.1034/j.1600-0749.2003.00032.x/abstract

13. Valia AK, Dutta PK. IADVL Text book and Atlas of Dermatology. Mumbai: Bhalani Publishing House; 2001. p. 608.

14. Number of people (all ages) living with HIV. Estimates by WHO region. 2016. http://apps.who.int/gho/data/view.main.22100WHO?lang=en

15. Aetna. Insurance Policy. "Aetna considers treatments for vitiligo cosmetic if they do not affect the underlying condition and do not result in improved protection against skin cancer." Accessed on November 1, 2017. http://www.aetna.com/cpb/medical/data/400_499/0422.html

16. Dumas-Mallet E, Smith A, Boraud T, Gonon F. 2017. Poor replication validity of biomedical association studies reported by newspapers. PLoS ONE12(2): e0172650. https://doi.org/10.1371/journal.pone.0172650

17. Silverberg N. Pediatric vitiligo. Pediatr Clin North Am. 2014 Apr;61(2):347-66. doi: 10.1016/j.pcl.2013.11.008. https://www.ncbi.nlm.nih.gov/pubmed/24636650

18. Ezzedine K, Silverberg N. A Practical Approach to the Diagnosis and Treatment of Vitiligo in Children. Pediatrics. 2016 Jul;138(1). pii: e20154126. doi: 10.1542/peds.2015-4126. https://www.ncbi.nlm.nih.gov/pubmed/27328922

19. Silverberg J, Silverberg N. Clinical features of vitiligo associated with comorbid autoimmune disease: a prospective survey. J Am Acad Dermatol. 2013

Nov;69(5):824-6. doi: 10.1016/j.jaad.2013.04.050.
https://www.ncbi.nlm.nih.gov/pubmed/24124820

20. Teulings HE, Overkamp M, Ceylan E, et al. Decreased risk of melanoma and nonmelanoma skin cancer in patients with vitiligo: a survey among 1307 patients and their partners. Br J Dermatol. 2013 Jan;168(1):162-71. doi: 10.1111/bjd.12111.
https://www.ncbi.nlm.nih.gov/pubmed/23136900

21. Nordlund JJ. Vitiligo: A review of some facts lesser known about depigmentation. Indian J Dermatol 2011. 56:180-9. Available from: http://www.e-ijd.org/text.asp?2011/56/2/180/80413

22. Spritz R, Andersen G. Dermatol Clin. 2017 Apr;35(2):245-255. doi: 10.1016/j.det.2016.11.013.
https://www.ncbi.nlm.nih.gov/pubmed/28317533

23. Jin Y, Andersen G, Spritz R, et al. Genome-wide association studies of autoimmune vitiligo identify 23 new risk loci and highlight key pathways and regulatory variants. Nature Genetics 48, 1418–1424. 2016. doi:10.1038/ng.3680
https://www.nature.com/articles/ng.3680

24. Konigsberg E. Inside 'Mad Men': A Fine Madness. Rolling Stone magazine. September, 2010
http://www.rollingstone.com/movies/news/inside-mad-men-a-fine-madness-20100916

25. Silverberg J, Silverberg N. Vitiligo disease triggers: psychological stressors preceding the onset of disease. Cutis. 2015. 95(5):255-62.
https://www.ncbi.nlm.nih.gov/pubmed/26057504

26. Vitiligo Q&A. VR Foundation. 2014.
http://vrfoundation.org/foundation/download-center

27. Vitiligo: A Step-By-Step Guide To Diagnosis, Treatment and Prophylaxis. VR Foundation. 2017. ISBN 978-1-3706001-6-8.

28. Rezaei N, Gavalas NG, Weetman AP, Kemp EH. Autoimmunity as an aetiological factor in vitiligo. J Eur Acad Dermatol Venereol. 2007. 21(7):865-76. https://www.ncbi.nlm.nih.gov/pubmed/17658994

29. Boyle EA, Li Y, Pritchard J. An Expanded View of Complex Traits: From Polygenic to Omnigenic. Cell. 2017. Volume 169, Issue 7, 1177–1186 http://dx.doi.org/10.1016/j.cell.2017.05.038

30. Retseck G. Suited Science: What Are the Odds of Drawing *That* Card? Scientific American. 2012. https://www.scientificamerican.com/article/bring-science-home-cards-odds-probability/

31. Hong CK, Lee MH, Jeong KH, Cha CI, Yeo SG. Clinical analysis of hearing levels in vitiligo patients. Eur J Dermatol. 2009.19(1):50-6. doi: 10.1684/ejd.2008.0563 https://www.ncbi.nlm.nih.gov/pubmed/19059822

32. Cowan CL Jr, Halder RM, Grimes PE, et al. Ocular disturbances in vitiligo. J Am Acad Dermatol. 1986. Jul;15(1):17-24. https://www.ncbi.nlm.nih.gov/pubmed/3722505

33. Hercogová J, Schwartz RA, Lotti TM. Classification of vitiligo: a challenging endeavor. Dermatol Ther. 2012; 25 Suppl 1:S10-6. doi: 10.1111/dth.12010. https://www.ncbi.nlm.nih.gov/pubmed/23237033

34. Taïeb A, Picardo M; VETF Members. The definition and assessment of vitiligo: a consensus report of the Vitiligo European Task Force. Pigment Cell Res. 2007. 20(1):27-35. https://www.ncbi.nlm.nih.gov/pubmed/17250545

35. Attili VR, Attili SK. Segmental and Generalized Vitiligo: Both Forms Demonstrate Inflammatory Histopathological Features and Clinical Mosaicism. Indian J Dermatol. 2013 Nov-Dec.; 58(6): 433–438. doi: 10.4103/0019-5154.119949

36. Park JH, Lee DY. Segmental Vitiligo, Vitiligo - Management and Therapy, Dr. Kelly KyungHwa Park (Ed.) 2011. ISBN: 978-953-307-731-4, InTech, available from: http://www.intechopen.com/books/vitiligo-management-and-therapy/segmental-vitiligo

37. Silverberg JI, Reja M, Silverberg NB. Regional variation of and association of US birthplace with vitiligo extent. JAMA Dermatol. 2014 Dec;150(12):1298-305. https://www.ncbi.nlm.nih.gov/pubmed/25006795

38. The Koebner phenomenon is named after the German dermatologist Heinrich Koebner. It refers to the tendency of several skin conditions to affect areas after a skin trauma. The amount of trauma required can be very small, like a bruise, cut, minor burn, vaccination or tattoo.

39. Vitiligo Questionnaire by VR Foundation. 2014. http://vitinomics.net

40. Gupta LK, Singhi MK. Wood's lamp. Indian J Dermatol Venereol Leprol 2004;70:131-5 http://www.ijdvl.com/text.asp?2004/70/2/131/6915

41. Silverberg JI, Silverberg NB. False "highlighting" with Wood's lamp. Pediatr Dermatol. 2014 Jan-Feb;31(1):109-10. doi: 10.1111/j.1525-1470.2012.01787.x. https://www.ncbi.nlm.nih.gov/pubmed/22747772

42. Biswas A, Chaudhari P, Julka PK, Rath GK. Radiation induced depigmentation disorder in two patients with breast cancer: Exploring a rare accompaniment. In Journal of the Egyptian National Cancer Institute, Volume 27, Issue 2, 2015, Pages 101-104. https://doi.org/10.1016/j.jnci.2015.01.003.

43. Silverberg JI, Silverberg NB. Vitiligo disease triggers: psychological stressors preceding the onset of disease. Cutis. 2015 May;95(5):255-62. https://www.ncbi.nlm.nih.gov/pubmed/26057504

44. Winter Consensus Conference in historic Kitzbühel, Austria. Under the chairmanship of Prof. Robert Schwartz participants have covered the broad spectrum of issues related to vitiligo, from genetics to efficiency of various experimental treatments and "soon to be introduced" treatments. Attendees were inspired by Nobel Laureates: Kurt Wüthrich's lecture on a multi-disciplinary structural biology approach, and by Charles H. Townes' one emphasizing the compatibility of science and religion. http://vrfoundation.org/researchers--3/collaboration/vitiligo-workshops/roundtable-on-vitiligo

45. Yue E, Bai H, Lian L, et al. Effect of chloride on the formation of volatile disinfection byproducts in chlorinated swimming pools. In Water Research. 2016. Volume 105, Pages 413-420. http://www.sciencedirect.com/science/article/pii/S0043135416306959

46. Vine K, Meulener M, Shieh S, Silverberg NB. Vitiliginous lesions induced by amyl nitrite exposure. Cutis. 2013 Mar;91(3):129-36. https://www.ncbi.nlm.nih.gov/pubmed/23617083

47. Contact Allergen Database provides information to the more common causes of allergic contact dermatitis.http://contactallergy.com

48. The Household Products Database of the U.S. National Library of Medicine links over 18,000 consumer brands to health effects from Safety Data Sheets. https://householdproducts.nlm.nih.gov/index.htm

49. Vine K, Meulener M, Shieh S, Silverberg NB. Cutis. 2013 Mar;91(3):129-36. https://www.ncbi.nlm.nih.gov/pubmed/23617083

50. Rogers C, King D, Chadha L, Kothandapani JSG. 'Black Henna Tattoo': art or allergen? BMJ Case Reports. 2016; doi:10.1136/bcr-2015-212232 http://casereports.bmj.com/content/2016/bcr-2015-212232.full

51. Scientific Committee on Consumer Safety Opinion On p-Phenylenediamine. 2012. http://ec.europa.eu/health/scientific_committees/consumer_safety/docs/sccs_o_094.pdf

52. David Tan. Who's The Fairest Of Them All? Asian Scientist Magazine. 2012. http://www.asianscientist.com/2012/09/features/skin-whitening-products-asia-2012/

53. World Health Organization. Mercury in skin lightening products. 2011. http://www.who.int/ipcs/assessment/public_health/mercury_flyer.pdf

54. Kanebo. Update regarding voluntary recall in Japan of products containing the quasi-drug ingredient "Rhododenol" and Kanebo's Response. 2013. http://www.kanebo.com/pressroom/pressrelease/20130723.pdf

55. The DrugBank is a unique bioinformatics and cheminformatics resource that combines detailed drug data with comprehensive drug target information. Database version 5.0.9, released 2017-10-02. https://www.drugbank.ca

56. Tufts Center for the Study of Drug Development. Cost to Develop and Win Marketing Approval for a New Drug Is $2.6 Billion. November 2014. http://csdd.tufts.edu/news/complete_story/pr_tufts_csdd_2014_cost_study

57. Graham JR. The National Center For Policy Analysis.

The Crisis in Drug Research and Development. March 2015. http://www.ncpa.org/pub/ib158

58. Matthew Herper. The Cost Of Creating A New Drug Now $5 Billion, Pushing Big Pharma To Change. Forbes, August 2013. https://www.forbes.com/sites/matthewherper/2013/08/11/how-the-staggering-cost-of-inventing-new-drugs-is-shaping-the-future-of-medicine/#3f04d38213c3

59. Life SciVC. Blog of Bruce Booth, an early stage venture capitalist, writer, researcher. http://lifescivc.com/wp-content/uploads/2014/11/Cost-of-Drug-RD_Nov2014.xlsx

60. Booth B. A Billion Here, A Billion There: The Cost Of Making A Drug Revisited. Forbes, November 2014. https://www.forbes.com/sites/brucebooth/2014/11/21/a-billion-here-a-billion-there-the-cost-of-making-a-drug-revisited/#759c42dc26a8

61. Kesselheim AS, Avorn J, Sarpatwari J. The High Cost of Prescription Drugs in the United States Origins and Prospects for Reform. JAMA. 2016;316(8):858-871. doi:10.1001/jama.2016.11237

62. Radtke MA, Schäfer I, Gajur A, et al. Willingness-to-pay and quality of life in patients with vitiligo. Br J Dermatol. 2009 Jul;161(1):134-9. doi: 10.1111/j.1365-2133.2009.09091.x. https://www.ncbi.nlm.nih.gov/pubmed/19298268

63. VR Foundation. Quick poll results: Cost of Vitiligo Treatments. 2016. http://vrfoundation.org/pages/quick-poll-results-cost-of-vitiligo-treatments

64. The global resource for scientific evidence in animal research: http://www.animalresearch.info/en/medical-advances/nobel-prizes/

65. Bergers LIJC, Reijnders CMA [...] Gibbs S. Immune-competent human skin disease models. Drug Discov

Today. 2016 Sep;21(9):1479-1488. doi:
10.1016/j.drudis.2016.05.008.
https://www.ncbi.nlm.nih.gov/pubmed/27265772

66. Boissy RE, Lamoreux ML. Animal models of an
acquired pigmentary disorder--vitiligo. Prog Clin Biol
Res. 1988;256:207-18
https://www.ncbi.nlm.nih.gov/pubmed/3285351

67. Essien IE, Harris JE. Erratum to "Animal Models of
Vitiligo: Matching the Model to the Question"
Dermatologica Sinica, Volume 33, Issue 1, March 2015,
Pages 47. https://doi.org/10.1016/j.dsi.2014.09.008

68. Singh VP, Motiani RK, Gokhale RS, et al. Water
Buffalo (Bubalus bubalis) as a spontaneous animal
model of Vitiligo. Pigment Cell Melanoma Res. 2016
Jul;29(4):465-9. doi: 10.1111/pcmr.12485.
https://www.ncbi.nlm.nih.gov/pubmed/27124831

69. Buranyi S. Is the staggeringly profitable business of
scientific publishing bad for science?
https://www.theguardian.com/science/2017/jun/27/profi
table-business-scientific-publishing-bad-for-science

70. Sci-Hub is a website with over 62 million academic
papers and articles available for direct download.
https://en.wikipedia.org/wiki/Sci-Hub

71. In solidarity with Library Genesis and Sci-Hub. 2015.
http://custodians.online

72. The name is derived from the meme *I Can Has
Cheezburger?*. It was started by scientist and behavior
therapist Dr. Andrea Kuszewski in 2011.

73. Gardner CC, Gardner JG. Bypassing Interlibrary Loan
Via Twitter: An Exploration of #icanhazpdf Requests.
The published PDF version of a contributed paper for
the Association of College and Research Libraries
(ACRL) 2015 conference in Portland, Oregon, can be
found at:

http://www.ala.org/acrl/sites/ala.org.acrl/files/content/conferences/confsandpreconfs/2015/Gardner.pdf

74. Open Payments Data: Find Your Doctor's Payments. https://openpaymentsdata.cms.gov

75. Estimating the reproducibility of psychological science, by Open Science Collaboration. Science Aug 2015. Vol. 349, Issue 6251, aac4716; DOI: 10.1126/science.aac4716. http://science.sciencemag.org/content/349/6251/aac4716

76. Clinical Trials Registration and Results Information Submission. National Institutes of Health, Department of Health and Human Services. January 2017. https://s3.amazonaws.com/public-inspection.federalregister.gov/2016-22129.pdf

77. Sumner P, Chambers CD, et al. The association between exaggeration in health related science news and academic press releases: retrospective observational study. BMJ. 2014. 349:g7015 http://www.bmj.com/content/349/bmj.g7015

78. Ioannidis JPA. The Mass Production of Redundant, Misleading, and Conflicted Systematic Reviews and Meta-analyses. The Milbank Quarterly, Vol. 94, No. 3, 2016 (pp. 485-514) https://www.milbank.org/wp-content/files/documents/The_Mass_Production_of_Redundant_Misleading_and_Conflicted_Systematic_Reviews_and_Meta-Analyses.pdf

79. The Fitzpatrick Skin Type is a skin classification system first developed by Harvard Medical School dermatologist Thomas B. Fitzpatrick in 1975.

80. Whitton M, Pinart M, Batchelor, et al. 2016. Evidence-based management of vitiligo: summary of a Cochrane systematic review. Br J Dermatol, 174: 962–969. doi:10.1111/bjd.14356 http://onlinelibrary.wiley.com/doi/10.1111/bjd.14356/full/

81. Famous Vitiligans. Many celebrities have dealt with vitiligo while remaining in the public eye, maintaining a positive outlook, and having a successful career. Here are a few famous and courageous people who show that vitiligo doesn't have to get in the way of your hopes and dreams: http://vrfoundation.org/patients--2/famous-vitiligans

82. Bae JM, Jung HM, Hong BY, et al. Phototherapy for VitiligoA Systematic Review and Meta-analysis. *JAMA Dermatol.* 2017;153(7):666–674. doi:10.1001/jamadermatol.2017.0002 https://jamanetwork.com/journals/jamadermatology/article-abstract/2612724? widget=personalizedcontent&previousarticle=479293

83. Esmat S, Hegazy RA, Shalaby S, et al. Phototherapy and Combination Therapies for Vitiligo. Dermatol Clin. 2017 Apr;35(2):171-192. doi: 10.1016/j.det.2016.11.008. https://www.ncbi.nlm.nih.gov/pubmed/28317527

84. Grimes DR, Robbins C, O'Hare NJ. Dose modeling in ultraviolet phototherapy. Med Phys. 2010 Oct;37(10):5251-7. http://onlinelibrary.wiley.com/doi/10.1118/1.3484093/abstract

85. Scherschun L, Kim JJ, Lim HW. Narrow-band ultraviolet B is a useful and well-tolerated treatment for vitiligo. J Am Acad Dermatol 2001;44:999-1003 http://dx.doi.org/10.1067/mjd.2001.114752

86. Bhatnagar A, Kanwar AJ, Parsad D. Comparison of systemic PUVA and NB-UVB in the treatment of vitiligo: an open prospective study. Journal of the European Academy of Dermatology and Venereology, 2007: 638–642. doi:10.1111/j 1468-3083.2006. 02035.x http://onlinelibrary.wiley.com/doi/10.1111/j.1468-3083.2006.02035.x/abstract

87. Mohammad TF, Hamzavi IH, Harris JE, et al. The Vitiligo Working Group recommendations for narrowband ultraviolet B light phototherapy treatment of vitiligo. Presented at PigmentaryCon 2016, April 2, 2016, Delhi, India. J Am Acad Dermatol 2017;76,5:879-888
http://dx.doi.org/10.1016/j.jaad.2016.12.041

88. Park KKH, Murase JE. Ultraviolet B (UVB) Phototherapy in the Treatment of Vitiligo, Vitiligo - Management and Therapy. Dr. Kelly KyungHwa Park (Ed.) 2011. ISBN: 978-953-307-731-4, InTech
http://cdn.intechopen.com/pdfs-wm/24970.pdf

89. Speeckaert R, van Geel N. Vitiligo: An Update on Pathophysiology and Treatment Options. Am J Clin Dermatol. 2017 Jun 2. doi: 10.1007/s40257- 017-0298-5.
https://www.ncbi.nlm.nih.gov/pubmed/28577207

90. Taïeb A, Seneschal J, Mazereeuw-Hautier J. Special Considerations in Children with Vitiligo. Dermatol Clin. 2017 Apr;35(2):229-233. doi: 10.1016/j.det.2016.11.011.
https://www.ncbi.nlm.nih.gov/pubmed/28317531

91. Anbar TS, Westerhof W, Abdel-Rahman AT, El-Khayyat MA. Evaluation of the effects of NB-UVB in both segmental and non-segmental vitiligo affecting different body sites. Photodermatology, Photoimmunology & Photomedicine, 22: 157–163. doi: 10.1111/j.1600-0781.2006.00222.x
http://onlinelibrary.wiley.com/wol1/doi/10.1111/j.1600-0781.2006.00222.x/full

92. Kanwar AJ, Dogra S. Narrow-band UVB for the treatment of generalized vitiligo in children. Clinical and Experimental Dermatology, 30: 332–336. doi: 10.1111/j.1365-2230.2005.01837.x
http://onlinelibrary.wiley.com/doi/10.1111/j.1365-2230.2005.01837.x/full/

93. Van Driessche F, Silverberg N. Current Management of Pediatric Vitiligo. Paediatr Drugs. 2015 Aug;17(4):303-13. doi: 10.1007/s40272-015-0135-3. https://www.ncbi.nlm.nih.gov/pubmed/26022363

94. Harris JE, Scharf M. Vitiligo nbUVB Treatment Protocol. Available at: https://www.umassmed.edu/globalassets/vitiligo/umas s-uvb-phototherapy-guidelines.pdf

95. Mysore V, Shashikumar B M. Targeted phototherapy. Indian J Dermatol Venereol Leprol 2016;82:1-6. http://www.ijdvl.com/text.asp?2016/82/1/1/172902

96. Spencer JM, Nossa R, Ajmeri J. Treatment of vitiligo with the 308-nm excimer laser: A pilot study. J Am Acad Dermatol 2002;46:727-31 http://dx.doi.org/10.1067/mjd.2002.121357

97. Photoaging is a premature aging of the skin due to its prolonged exposure to UV light from the sun, phototherapy equipment or tanning beds. Photoaging causes skin changes that include fine and deep wrinkles, scars, irregular pigmentation, freckles, leathery texture, and sagging in areas exposed to the sun. Its effects can appear starting from teens and early twenties. Once photoaging has started, it's hard to reverse. Photoaging can be minimized by adopting simple sun protection habits: graded sun exposure, sunscreen, and protective clothing. Most photoaging treatments aim to increase firmness and elasticity of photodamaged skin.

98. Gilchrest BA. Photoaging. Journal of Investigative Dermatology. July 2013.Volume 133, Supplement 2, Pages E2–E6 http://www.jidonline.org/article/S0022-202X(15)41893-7/fulltext

99. Moriwaki S, Takahashi Y. Photoaging and DNA repair.

J Dermatol Sci. 2008;50(3):169-76.
https://www.ncbi.nlm.nih.gov/pubmed/17920816

100. Eleftheriadou V, Thomas K, Ravenscroft J, et al.
Feasibility, double-blind, randomised, placebo-
controlled, multi-centre trial of hand-held NB-UVB
phototherapy for the treatment of vitiligo at home (HI-
Light trial: Home Intervention of Light therapy).
Trials. 2014 Feb 8;15:51. doi: 10.1186/1745-6215-15-51.
https://www.ncbi.nlm.nih.gov/pubmed/24507484

101. Wind BS, Wolkerstorfer A, et al. Home vs. outpatient
narrowband ultraviolet B therapy for the treatment of
nonsegmental vitiligo: a retrospective questionnaire
study. Br J Dermatol. 2010 May;162(5):1142-4. doi:
10.1111/j.1365-2133.2010.09678.x.
https://www.ncbi.nlm.nih.gov/pubmed/20199553

102. Rajpara AN, O'Neill JL, Nolan BV, et al. UC Davis
Dermatology Online Journal 2010. 16 (12): 2
https://escholarship.org/uc/item/2ts6s057

103. National Managed Clinical Network for Phototherapy
in Scotland is a supervised home phototherapy service
for those who cannot regularly attend hospital
units. http://www.photonet.scot.nhs.uk/professionals-
area/home-phototherapy/

104. Lim HW, Silpa-archa N, Lebwohl M, et al.
Phototherapy in dermatology: A call for action. J Am
Acad Dermatol 2015. 72;6:1078-1080
http://dx.doi.org/10.1016/j.jaad.2015.03.017

105. From the company's press-release: "Clarify's
technologies are designed to allow physicians to
control treatment and assess patient progress
remotely." https://venturebeat.com/2017/10/12/clarify-
medical-and-dermatologistoncall-announce-a-
partnership-to-innovate-the-treatment-of-chronic-
skin-conditions/

106. For all USA shipments of phototherapy devices, a prescription is required by law per US Code of Federal Regulations 21CFR801.109 "Prescription Devices". Not just a dermatologist but any registered General Practitioner, Medical Doctor or Nurse Practitioner can write a prescription as (a) traditional paper prescription, (b) letter on the on the physician's letterhead, or (c) use online forms provided by vendors of UVB phototherapy devices.

107. Koo J, Nakamura M. Prescribing a Home Phototherapy Booth. Clinical Cases in Phototherapy. Clinical Cases in Dermatology. Springer, Cham. 2017 https://doi.org/10.1007/978-3-319-51599-1_28

108. Gill L, Lim HW. Drug-Induced Photosensitivity. In: Hall J., Hall B. (eds) Cutaneous Drug Eruptions. Springer, London. 2015. https://doi.org/10.1007/978-1-4471-6729-7_10

109. Levine IJ. Medications That Increase Sensitivity To Light. U.S. Department of Health and Human Services. 1990. https://www.fda.gov/downloads/Radiation-EmittingProducts/RadiationEmittingProductsandProc edures/SurgicalandTherapeutic/UCM135813.pdf

110. Hashizume H. Skin aging and dry skin. J. Dermatol. 2004;31:603–609. doi: 10.1111/j.1346-8138.2004.tb00565.x. https://www.ncbi.nlm.nih.gov/pubmed/15492432

111. Shin J, Kim JE, Lee KW et al. A Combination of Soybean and Haematococcus Extract Alleviates Ultraviolet B-Induced Photoaging. Int J Mol Sci. 2017 Mar 22;18(3). pii: E682. doi: 10.3390/ijms18030682. https://www.ncbi.nlm.nih.gov/pubmed/28327532

112. Sitek J, Loeb M, Ronnevig J. 2007. Narrowband UVB therapy for vitiligo: does the repigmentation last? Journal of the European Academy of Dermatology

and Venereology, 21: 891–896. doi:10.1111/j.1468-3083.2007.01980.x
http://onlinelibrary.wiley.com/doi/10.1111/j.1468-3083.2007.01980.x/abstract

113. Cavalie M, Ezzedine K, Passeron T, et al. Maintenance Therapy of Adult Vitiligo with 0.1% Tacrolimus Ointment: A Randomized, Double Blind, Placebo–Controlled Study. Journal of Investigative Dermatology (2015) 135, 970–974; doi:10.1038/jid.2014.527.
http://www.jidonline.org/article/S0022-202X(15)37181-5/pdf

114. Speeckaert R, van Geel N. Vitiligo: An Update on Pathophysiology and Treatment Options. Am J Clin Dermatol. June 2017. https://doi.org/10.1007/s40257-017-0298-5

115. Taieb A, Alomar A, Picardo M and the writing group of the Vitiligo European Task Force (VETF) in cooperation with the European Academy of Dermatology and Venereology (EADV) and the Union Européenne des Médecins Spécialistes (UEMS) (2013), Guidelines for the management of vitiligo: the European Dermatology Forum consensus. British Journal of Dermatology, 168: 5–19. doi:10.1111/j.1365-2133.2012.11197.x
http://onlinelibrary.wiley.com/wol1/resolve/doi?DOI=10.1111/j.1365-2133.2012.11197.x

116. Gianfaldoni S, Zanardelli M, Lotti T. Vitiligo Repigmentation: What's New? J Dermatolog Clin Res. 2014. 2(3): 1023.
https://www.jscimedcentral.com/Dermatology/dermatology-2-1023.pdf

117. Ho N, Pope E, Weinstein M, et al. A double-blind, randomized, placebo-controlled trial of topical

tacrolimus 0·1% vs. clobetasol propionate 0·05% in childhood vitiligo. British Journal of Dermatology, 2011. 165: 626–632. doi:10.1111/j.1365-2133.2011.10351.x http://onlinelibrary.wiley.com/doi/10.1111/j.1365-2133.2011.10351.x/abstract

118. Gawkrodger DG, Ormerod AD, Young K, et al. Vitiligo: concise evidence based guidelines on diagnosis and management. Postgraduate Medical Journal 2010;86:466-471. http://dx.doi.org/10.1136/pgmj.2009.093278

119. Lotti T, Buggiani G, Hercogova J. Targeted and combination treatments for vitiligo. Comparative evaluation of different current modalities in 458 subjects. 2008. Dermatologic Therapy, 21: S20–S26. doi:10.1111/j.1529-8019.2008.00198.x http://onlinelibrary.wiley.com/doi/10.1111/j.1529-8019.2008.00198.x/abstract

120. Nordal EJ, Guleng GE, Rönnevig JR. Treatment of vitiligo with narrowband-UVB (TL01) combined with tacrolimus ointment (0.1%) vs. placebo ointment, a randomized right/left double-blind comparative study. Journal of the European Academy of Dermatology and Venereology. 2011. 25: 1440–1443. doi:10.1111/j.1468-3083.2011.04002.x http://onlinelibrary.wiley.com/doi/10.1111/j.1468-3083.2011.04002.x/abstract

121. Ramaiah et al. A Double Blind Randomized Phase IV Clinical Trial of basic Fibroblast Growth Factor Related Deca-peptide in Vitiligo. Pigmentary Disorders 2015, S3:1 http://dx.doi.org/10.4172/2376-0427.S3-004

122. NEOVIR® (Sodium Oxodihydroacridinylacetate): Press Release, Abstract and Presentation can be accessed at VR Foundation website:

http://vrfoundation.org/pages/sodium-oxodihydroacridinylacetate

123. Korobko IV, Lomonosov KM. Acridone acetic acid, sodium salt, as an agent to stop vitiligo progression: a pilot study. Dermatol Ther. 2014 Jul-Aug;27(4):219-22. doi: 10.1111/dth.12121. https://www.ncbi.nlm.nih.gov/pubmed/24548590

124. Pasricha JS, Seetharam KA, Dashore A. Evaluation of Five Different Regimes For the Treatment of Vitiligo. Indian J Dermatol Venereol Leprol. 1989 Jan-Feb;55(1):18-21. https://www.ncbi.nlm.nih.gov/pubmed/28112107

125. Parsad D, Gupta S. Standard guidelines of care for vitiligo surgery. Indian J Dermatol Venereol Leprol 2008;74, Suppl S1:37-45. http://www.ijdvl.com/text.asp?2008/74/7/37/42286

126. Check out World Vitiligo Map for contact information: www.VRFoundation.org/maps/all

127. Pizzoccaro A, Perra A., Lotti T. Low Dose Medicine: The New Paradigm. Innovative Therapies in Dermatology. 2015. Guna S.p.a. Available from: https://guna.com/wp-content/uploads/2015/12/Brochure-Dermatologia-versione-Settembre-2015.pdf

128. Lotti T, Hercogova J, Tchernev G, et al. Vitiligo: successful combination treatment based on oral low dose cytokines and different topical treatments. J Biol Regul Homeost Agents. 2015 Jan-Mar;29(1 Suppl):53-8. https://www.ncbi.nlm.nih.gov/pubmed/26016984

129. Rothstein B, Joshipura D, Rosmarin D, et al. Treatment of vitiligo with the topical Janus kinase inhibitor ruxolitinib. Journal of the American Academy of Dermatology, Volume 76 , Issue 6 , 1054 - 1060.e1 http://dx.doi.org/10.1016/j.jaad.2017.02.049

130. Lim HW, Grimes PE, Lebwohl M, et al. Afamelanotide and narrowband UV-B phototherapy for the treatment of vitiligo: a randomized multicenter trial. JAMA Dermatol. 2015 Jan;151(1):42-50. doi: 10.1001/jamadermatol.2014.1875. https://www.ncbi.nlm.nih.gov/pubmed/25230094

131. Therapy For Vitiligo. Patent US 9,801,924 B2. Date of patent October 31, 2017. http://www.sharescene.com/index.php?act=attach&type=post&id=48600

132. ClinicalTrials.gov is a database of privately and publicly funded clinical studies conducted around the world. This resource is provided by the U.S. National Library of Medicine. https://clinicaltrials.gov

133. Buser GL, Mató S, Zhang AY, et al. *Notes from the Field:* Late-Onset Infant Group B Streptococcus Infection Associated with Maternal Consumption of Capsules Containing Dehydrated Placenta — Oregon, 2016. MMWR Morb Mortal Wkly Rep. 2017. 66:677–678. http://dx.doi.org/10.15585/mmwr.mm6625a4

134. Miyares CM, Barca IH, Miyares ED, González AP. Efectividad de un extracto de placenta humana con Calcio (Melagenina Plus) en el tratamiento del Vitiligo. Revista Cubana de Investigaciones Biomédicas 2009;28(3):9-24 http://scieloprueba.sld.cu/pdf/ibi/v28n3/ibi02309.pdf

135. Bedi MK, Shenefelt PD. Herbal Therapy in Dermatology. Arch Dermatol. 2002;138(2):232-242. doi:10.1001/archderm.138.2.232 http://jamanetwork.com/journals/jamadermatology/fullarticle/1105343

136. Ernst E. Adverse effects of herbal drugs in dermatology. British Journal of Dermatology. 2000. 143: 923–929. doi:10.1046/j.1365-2133.2000.03822.x

http://onlinelibrary.wiley.com/doi/10.1046/j.1365-2133.2000.03822.x/abstract

137. Smith N, Shin DB, Brauer JA, et al. Use of complementary and alternative medicine among adults with skin disease: results from a national survey. J Am Acad Dermatol. 2009 Mar;60(3):419-25. doi: 10.1016/j.jaad.2008.11.905 https://www.ncbi.nlm.nih.gov/pubmed/19157642

138. McFadden R, Peterson N. Interactions between drugs and four common medicinal herbs. Nurs Stand. 2011 Jan 12-18;25(19):65-8. https://www.ncbi.nlm.nih.gov/pubmed/21287929

139. Ayahuasca – also known as natem, ayawaska, iowaska or yage – is an Amazonian plant mixture that is capable of inducing altered states of consciousness. The word *ayahuasca* has been variously translated as "liana of the soul" or "liana of the dead." This is a brew made out of Banisteriopsis caapi vine and number of other ingredients, using a ritual process that lasts about 12 hours. The psychoactive effects last between 4 to 8 hours after ingestion, ranging from mildly stimulating to extremely visionary – somewhat similar to wearing an augmented reality headset. It is for this reason that *ayahuasca should be tried only in the presence of an experienced healer, or shaman.*

140. Nestor M, Bucay V, Waldorf H, et al. Polypodium leucotomos as an Adjunct Treatment of Pigmentary Disorders. J Clin Aesthet Dermatol. 2014 Mar;7(3):13-7. https://www.ncbi.nlm.nih.gov/pubmed/24688621

141. Moreira CG, Carrenho LZ, Otuki MF, et al. Pre-clinical evidences of Pyrostegia venusta in the treatment of vitiligo. J Ethnopharmacol. 2015 Jun 20;168:315-25. doi: 10.1016/j.jep.2015.03.080.

https://www.ncbi.nlm.nih.gov/pubmed/?
term=25862965

142. Saper RB, Kales SN, Paquin J. Heavy Metal Content of Ayurvedic Herbal Medicine Products. *JAMA*. 2004 ;292(23):2868-2873. doi:10.1001/jama.292.23.2868 https://jamanetwork.com/journals/jama/fullarticle/110 8395

143. Gao C, Yang L, Chen M, Zhang H. Principles of Differentiation and Prescription for Vitiligo in Traditional Chinese Medicine Based on a Literature Investigation. Integr Med Int 2015;2:149-156 https://doi.org/10.1159/000441845

144. Ko RJ. Adulterants in Asian Patent Medicines. N Engl J Med 1998; 339:847September 17, 1998DOI: 10.1056/NEJM199809173391214 http://www.nejm.org/doi/full/10.1056/NEJM1998091733 91214

145. Coghlan ML, Haile J, Moolhuijzen P, et al. Deep Sequencing of Plant and Animal DNA Contained within Traditional Chinese Medicines Reveals Legality Issues and Health Safety Concerns. PLoS Genet8(4): e1002657. 2012. https://doi.org/10.1371/journal.pgen.1002657

146. Parsad D, Pandhi R, Juneja A. Effectiveness of oral Ginkgo biloba in treating limited, slowly spreading vitiligo. Clin Exp Dermatol. 2003 May;28(3):285-7.n https://www.ncbi.nlm.nih.gov/pubmed/12780716

147. Szczurko O, Shear N, Taddio A, Boon H. Ginkgo biloba for the treatment of vitilgo vulgaris: an open label pilot clinical trial. BMC Complement Altern Med. 2011; 11: 21. doi: 10.1186/1472-6882-11-21 https://www.ncbi.nlm.nih.gov/pmc/articles/PMC30654 45/

148. Unger M. Pharmacokinetic drug interactions involving

Ginkgo biloba. Drug Metab Rev. 2013 Aug;45(3):353-85.
doi: 10.3109/03602532.2013.815200.
https://www.ncbi.nlm.nih.gov/pubmed/23865865

149. Rietjens IM, Boersma MG, Koeman JH, et al. The pro-oxidant chemistry of the natural antioxidants vitamin C, vitamin E, carotenoids and flavonoids. Environmental Toxicology and Pharmacology. Volume 11, Issues 3-4, July 2002, Pages 321-333 https://doi.org/10.1016/S1382-6689(02)00003-0

150. Podmore ID, Griffiths HR, Herbert KE, et al. Vitamin C exhibits pro-oxidant properties. Nature. 1998 Apr 9;392(6676):559. https://www.ncbi.nlm.nih.gov/pubmed/9560150/

151. Kripke C. Is Oral Vitamin B_{12} as Effective as Intramuscular Injection? Am Fam Physician. 2006 Jan 1;73(1):65. http://gut.bmj.com/content/gutjnl/30/12/1686.full.pdf

152. T. Czarnowicki T, Harari M, Ruzicka T, Ingber A. Dead Sea climatotherapy for vitiligo: a retrospective study of 436 patients. Journal of the European Academy of Dermatology and Venereology. 2011. Volume 25, Issue 8, pages 959–963. http://onlinelibrary.wiley.com/doi/10.1111/j.1468-3083.2010.03903.x/abstract

153. Schallreuter KU, Moore J, Harari M, et al. Rapid initiation of repigmentation in vitiligo with Dead Sea climatotherapy in combination with pseudocatalase (PC-KUS). International Journal of Dermatology 2002, 41: 482–487. doi:10.1046/j.1365-4362.2002.01463.x http://onlinelibrary.wiley.com/doi/10.1046/j1365-4362.2002.01463.x/abstract

154. Gawkrodger DJ. Pseudocatalase and narrowband ultraviolet B for vitiligo: clearing the picture. Br J Dermatol. 2009 Oct;161(4):721-2. doi: 10.1111/j.1365-

2133.2009.09292.x.
https://www.ncbi.nlm.nih.gov/pubmed/19780755

155. Harari M. Climatotherapy of Skin Diseases at the Dead Sea – an update. Anales de Hidrología Médica. ISSN: 1887-0813 2012, Vol. 5, Núm. 1, 39-51 http://dx.doi.org/10.5209/rev_ANHM.2012.v5.n1.39168

156. Methods Of Vitiligo Treatment. A Collective Monograph. ISBN 978-601-80599-3-3. Almaty, Kazakhstan. 2016.

157. Rajatanavin N, Suwanachote S, Kulkollakarn S. Dihydroxyacetone: a safe camouflaging option in vitiligo. Int J Dermatol. 2008 Apr;47(4):402-6. doi: 10.1111/j.1365-4632.2008.03356.x. https://www.ncbi.nlm.nih.gov/pubmed/18377610

158. Zanderm is a convenient concealer lovingly made specifically for people with vitiligo. https://zanderm.com

159. Levy LL, Emer JJ. Emotional benefit of cosmetic camouflage in the treatment of facial skin conditions: personal experience and review. Clin Cosmet Investig Dermatol. 2012; 5: 173–182. doi: 10.2147/CCID.S33860 https://www.ncbi.nlm.nih.gov/pmc/articles/PMC3496327/

160. Mee D, Wong BJF. Medical Makeup for Concealing Facial Scars. Facial Plastic Surgery Vol. 28 No. 5/2012 . ISSN 0736-6825. http://dx.doi.org/10.1055/s-0032-1325647

161. Gupta D, Kumari R, Thappa DM. Depigmentation therapies in vitiligo. Indian J Dermatol Venereol Leprol. 2012;78:49-58. http://www.ijdvl.com/text.asp?2012/78/1/49/90946

162. Bolognia JL, Lapia K, Somma S. Depigmentation therapy. Dermatologic Therapy, 2001;14: 29–34. doi:10.1046/j.1529-8019.2001.014001029.x

http://onlinelibrary.wiley.com/wol1/doi/10.1046/j.1529-8019.2001.014001029.x/abstract

163. Oakley AM. Rapid repigmentation after depigmentation therapy: Vitiligo treated with monobenzyl ether of hydroquinone. 1996. Australasian Journal of Dermatology, 37: 96–98. doi:10.1111/j.1440-0960.1996.tb01014.x http://onlinelibrary.wiley.com/doi/10.1111/j.1440-0960.1996.tb01014.x/abstract

164. Gandhi V, Verma P, Naik G. Exogenous ochronosis After Prolonged Use of Topical Hydroquinone (2%) in a 50-Year-Old Indian Female. Indian Journal of Dermatology. 2012;57(5):394-395. doi:10.4103/0019-5154.100498. https://www.ncbi.nlm.nih.gov/pmc/articles/PMC3482806/

165. Maurício Z, Carlos D' Apparecida Santos. Depigmentation therapy for generalized vitiligo with topical 88% phenol solution. Anais Brasileiros de Dermatologia, 2005. 80(4), 415-416. https://dx.doi.org/10.1590/S0365-05962005000400013

166. Savant SS, Shenoy S. Chemical peeling with phenol: For the treatment of stable vitiligo and alopecia areata. Indian J Dermatol Venereol Leprol 1999;65:93-8. http://www.ijdvl.com/text.asp?1999/65/2/93/4776

167. Majid I, Imran S. Depigmentation with Q-switched Nd:YAG laser in universal vitiligo: a long-term follow-up study of 4 years. Lasers Med Sci. 2017; 32: 851. https://doi.org/10.1007/s10103-017-2183-0

168. Komen L, Zwertbroek L, Burger SJ, et al. Q-switched laser depigmentation in vitiligo, most effective in active disease. Br J Dermatol. 2013 Dec;169(6):1246-51.

doi: 10.1111/bjd.12571.

https://www.ncbi.nlm.nih.gov/pubmed/23909405

169. Lai YC, Yew YW, Kennedy C, Schwartz RA. 2017. Vitiligo and depression: a systematic review and meta-analysis of observational studies. Br J Dermatol, 177: 708–718. doi:10.1111/bjd.15199

http://onlinelibrary.wiley.com/doi/10.1111/bjd.15199/full

170. Cotterill JA, Cunliffe WJ. Suicide in dermatological patients. Br J Dermatol. 1997 Aug;137(2):246-50.

https://www.ncbi.nlm.nih.gov/pubmed/9292074/